If at first you don't *conceive*

A Complete Guide to Infertility from One of the Nation's Leading Clinics

WILLIAM SCHOOLCRAFT, MD, HCLD
Director of the Colorado Center for Reproductive Medicine

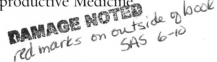

RODALE

To Cheri, Beau, and Michael

© 2010 by William Schoolcraft

Rodale books may be purchased for business or promotional use or for special sales. For information, please write to:
Special Markets Department, Rodale Inc.,
733 Third Avenue, New York, NY 10017.

Printed in the United States of America
Rodale Inc. makes every effort to use acid-free ∞, recycled paper ♻.

Book design by Christina Gaugler
Illustrations on pages 7, 10, 11, 71, 72, 88, 90, 94, 103, 163, 166, 168, 170, 217, 220, 221, and 222 by Echo Medical Media, 31586 Griffin Drive, Conifer, CO 80433
Graphs by Bill Youmans

Library of Congress Cataloging-in-Publication Data

Schoolcraft, William.
    If at first you don't conceive : a complete guide to infertility from one of the nation's leading clinics / William Schoolcraft.
        p.   cm.
    Includes index.
    ISBN-13: 978–1–60529–472–8 paperback
    ISBN-10: 1–60529–472–1 paperback
    1. Infertility—Popular works.   I. Title.
RC884.S36 2010
616.6'92—dc22   2009053966

Distributed to the trade by Macmillan

2   4   6   8   10   9   7   5   3   1   paperback

We inspire and enable people to improve their lives and the world around them
For more of our products visit rodalestore.com or call 800-848-4735

The following images were used with permission:

Contents

Part I: The Basics of What You Need to Know

Part II: The Most Common Fertility Challenges

Part III: The Most Common Solutions and Preventions

Part IV: Preserving Mind and Spirit

Part I

The Basics of What You Need to Know

CHAPTER ONE

Understanding
the Fertility Challenge

MY PATIENT TAYLOR was dedicated to her corporate career, but she always planned to have children someday. She never considered that there might be a problem. She never thought about *if* because her focus was always on *when*.

Yet when Taylor and her husband, Jared, decided that the time was right to start a family, they were unable to conceive. Taylor saw her infertility as a threat to the life she had envisioned. She fell into a depression that lasted more than 2 months.

For the first time in a life of considerable achievement, she felt defeated and out of control. She isolated herself from her friends and family, refusing to do anything but dwell on her thwarted desire to have a child.

Then, slowly, she pulled herself out of her despondency. Her intelligence and competitive nature came to the fore. Taylor resolved to fight for her fertility just as she fought for everything else she'd wanted.

As Taylor and millions of other women and men have discovered, the "fertility challenge" can be a bewildering, frustrating, and financially crippling experience. Too often, infertility patients give themselves over to physicians and treatment programs without understanding the science, the medicine, the odds or the economics. The fact is that at our clinic, we can help nearly 75 percent of the women who come to us become pregnant using quite traditional fertility treatments. And if a patient is willing to consider in vitro fertilization (IVF), egg donors, sperm donors, or surrogate mothers, the rate of conception moves much closer to 100 percent.

So there is hope, but men and women fighting infertility need to arm themselves with the latest medical science as well as commonsense practices to improve their chances. They need to become their own best advocates in their efforts to start a family.

Taylor discovered this when her initial series of treatments failed. After spending hundreds of thousands of dollars for treatments that did not result in pregnancy, she became determined to educate herself about infertility treatments—the science, the economics, and the best practitioners in the nation.

Taylor spent months immersed in research. Then she found her way to my clinic. In our initial discussions, Taylor's frustration and anger were obvious, but so was her determination. Still, she balked when I explained that I wanted to do an extensive series of initial tests, because she'd already gone through similar tests.

We insist on doing our own tests with each patient because too often we've found that we cannot rely on what has been done by other physicians and clinics. This proved true also in Taylor's case. We found that the "shells" around her eggs were much thicker than is normal, so the embryo could not break free and attach to the uterine lining.

Fortunately, we had worked with pioneering embryologist Jacques Cohen, PhD, whom one journalist described as "the IVF lab god." Dr. Cohen pioneered micromanipulation techniques for operating on eggs, sperm, and embryos. His work led to the development of assisted hatching, which promotes pregnancy by initiating the hatching process following fertilization.

Dr. Cohen observed that embryos with a thin shell had a higher rate of implantation during IVF. He deduced that making a tiny hole in the shell might help the embryo "hatch" and give it a better chance to implant in the uterus.

Assisted hatching, which has become a routine procedure, has been a boon for those whom other assisted reproductive procedures have failed, and also for older women. It also worked beautifully for Taylor. We took her through her fifth IVF cycle and she became pregnant—with twins.

More than *7.3 million* women and their partners in the United States are unable to have children because of infertility challenges, according to the American

Society for Reproductive Medicine. That figure represents nearly 12 percent of the nation's reproductive-age population.

There are many excellent clinics across the United States where you can seek top-notch treatment from fertility specialists. This book is based on the experiences and knowledge of our staff at the Colorado Center for Reproductive Medicine. Our clinic has consistently achieved annual birth rates that are among the highest in the United States, according to figures published by the Centers for Disease Control and Prevention (CDC) in Atlanta. It also was named as the nation's number one fertility clinic in a survey and data analysis published by *Child* magazine in 2005.

As astounding as it may seem, our clinic is responsible for the successful births of nearly 30,000 children over the past 20 years—most of them born to men and women who had been told that they might never experience the joys of parenthood. Because of our consistently high success rates, patients from more than 40 countries, facing every fertility challenge imaginable, come to our facility in the foothills of the Rocky Mountains. They come from a diverse mix of cultures, backgrounds, and professions.

Yet all too often they come to us burdened not only by infertility but also by inaccurate diagnoses, inadequate treatment, and a lack of the scientifically sound information they need to make intelligent and important decisions.

Women and men faced with infertility are hungry for up-to-date information and medically sound guidance. Their psychological stress has been shown to equal that of chronic pain victims, or those who are diagnosed with cancer or AIDS. The dropout rate for patients undergoing infertility treatment is well over 50 percent.

Infertility diagnoses and treatments can take months, and even years. That is why it is so important that women and men who are infertile have access to accurate and up to date information *before* they begin lengthy and costly treatments. Too often, desperate women and men seek treatment with a fertility specialist only after wasting crucial time either denying that they have a physical problem, or relying on the advice of someone who does not specialize in infertility. Many say that they wish they'd had a greater understanding of "how it all works" earlier in their fertility fights.

The medical science addressing infertility has taken tremendous leaps in the past 5 years. This book is designed to be a comprehensive, up-to-date guide for women and men who need to educate themselves so they don't waste precious time and deplete their financial resources fighting infertility. It provides the information and answers they need to make educated, thoughtful decisions—not decisions based on emotion—about the best treatments to pursue. As you begin your fertility fight, this book will provide you with vital information on:

○ Choosing the right physician and medical facility

○ Deciding which tests are most appropriate

○ Dealing with the emotional challenges of infertility

○ Understanding the financial aspects of treatment

○ Finding the latest proven treatments for each specific condition

○ Learning the latest success rates for each treatment

○ Working effectively with doctors and nurses

○ Fostering greater understanding between spouses and partners

It also provides up-to-date medical science and other helpful information in these key areas:

○ Fertility drugs

○ Insemination

○ In vitro fertilization

○ Egg and sperm donation

○ Gestational carriers (surrogates)

○ Male infertility treatments

○ Polycystic ovary syndrome

○ Endometriosis

○ Tubal and uterine conditions

○ Egg preservation through freezing

○ Fertility options for cancer patients

○ Fertility options for women over 40

○ Genetic testing and counseling

○ Acupuncture and other alternative approaches

This book offers guidance to help you identify your infertility issues and to help you ask the right questions in discussions with your medical team so you can work together to find the best solution for you to achieve your dream of having a baby.

Understanding Infertility

To understand infertility, you must first understand fertility and how human reproduction normally works. As an introduction to the rest of the book, let's look at the normal reproductive functions of males and females.

One key fact is that each woman is born with all of the eggs that she will ever produce. Amazingly, it is estimated that most female babies have more than a million eggs in their little bodies at birth. By the time puberty arrives, however, that number has decreased to about 300,000. Of these, only a few hundred will actually be released during a woman's reproductive years (see Figure 1).

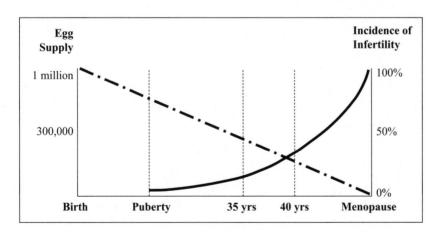

Figure 1: A woman's lifetime supply of eggs

The players in this complex cycle of female fertility include:

○ The *pituitary gland*, which produces follicle-stimulating hormone (FSH) and luteinizing hormone (LH)

○ The *ovary*, which produces the hormones estrogen and progesterone

○ The *follicle*, which contains the developing egg

○ The *fallopian tube*, where the sperm and egg meet and which transports the fertilized egg to the uterus

○ The *uterus*, which allows for implantation

Female fertility is rooted in the menstrual cycle, the time from the beginning of one period to the beginning of the next. A menstrual cycle begins with the onset of bleeding, or menses, caused by a fall in estrogen levels. This fall in estrogen causes a rise in FSH, which initiates the growth of a developing follicle. A follicle is a small, fluid-filled structure that contains the egg.

As the follicle continues to grow in size, it produces estrogen. This estrogen in turn stimulates the growth of the uterine lining, or endometrium. The endometrium increases from a very thin 1 to 2 millimeters to a thickness of 8 to 12 millimeters by the time of ovulation. At this thickness, the endometrium can support implantation or attachment of the embryo.

The follicle containing the egg continues to grow from a few millimeters up to a mean diameter of about 18 to 20 millimeters. At this point estrogen levels are elevated and as a result the endometrial lining is thickened and ready to receive the embryo.

The pituitary gland that has been directly controlling the growth of the follicle with FSH now secretes a burst of LH, which causes the follicle to rupture and release the egg from the ovary. The LH also causes the egg to undergo the process of maturation, and in this process, a genetic division of the chromosomes, called *meiosis*, occurs. During meiosis, the egg's 46 chromosomes are cut down to only 23 chromosomes. This prepares the egg for fertilization, when the sperm will enter the egg bearing its own 23-chromosome set. Together, the two sets of 23 chromosomes will yield an embryo with 46 chromosomes, the proper number for human development.

The LH surge also transforms the follicle—after its release of the egg—into a structure called the *corpus luteum*. The job of the corpus luteum is to not only

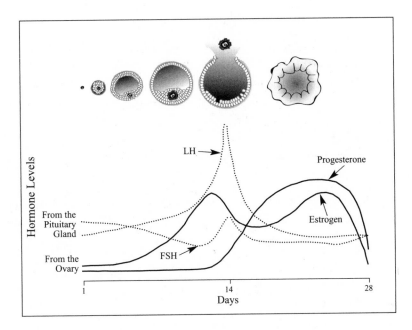

Figure 2: Changes across the menstrual cycle

continue manufacturing estrogen but also to begin producing progesterone. Progesterone transforms the uterine lining into a *secretory pattern* that will allow the endometrium to nourish the embryo, which in turn will allow the embryo to attach or implant into the uterine wall (see Figure 2).

Once ovulation occurs, the egg is captured by the *fimbria*, the finger-like structures at the end of the fallopian tube. *Cilia*, or hair-like structures inside the tube, beat in the same direction to propel the egg down the tube toward the uterus. It is at the entrance to the fallopian tube where the sperm meets the egg and the magic of fertilization occurs.

But the journey is far from over. After fertilization, the embryo takes a leisurely trip down the fallopian tube for 3 to 4 days, even as it is dividing into two cells, four cells, and so on, up to approximately 16 to 20 cells. At this stage, called the *morula stage*, the embryo leaves the fallopian tube and enters the uterus. By day 5 to 6 of growth, the embryo reaches a stage called the *blastocyst*. Remember that name, as it becomes an important aspect of the fertility challenge if something goes wrong (see Figure 3).

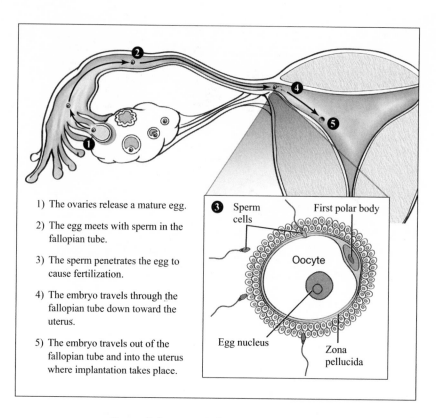

1) The ovaries release a mature egg.

2) The egg meets with sperm in the fallopian tube.

3) The sperm penetrates the egg to cause fertilization.

4) The embryo travels through the fallopian tube down toward the uterus.

5) The embryo travels out of the fallopian tube and into the uterus where implantation takes place.

Sperm cells

First polar body

Oocyte

Egg nucleus

Zona pellucida

Figure 3: From ovulation to implantation

At the blastocyst stage, the embryo is like an aircraft with two compartments. In first class is a group of cells called the *inner cell mass*, which are baby-makers. In coach class you'll find a group of cells called the *trophectoderm*, which will compose the placenta. These placenta or trophectoderm cells surround an inner, fluid-filled cavity called the *blastocele cavity*. It is at this stage that the embryo is ready to attach to the uterine wall. The blastocyst hatches out of its shell, which is called the *zona pellucida*, and attaches to the uterine lining. This process is called *implantation*—another term worth remembering.

The uterine lining has been pumped full of estrogen and progesterone, which are produced by the ovary to prepare for implantation. The ovary continues to make estrogen and progesterone for about 14 days from the time of ovulation. If a pregnancy begins, the embryo produces a hormone called *human chorionic gonadotropin,* or hCG, that signals the ovary to continue the production of estrogen and progesterone. These hormones help ensure that the uterine lining remains intact, thus allowing the embryo to maintain its growth. If there is no pregnancy, hCG is not produced, and 14 days after ovulation, estrogen and progesterone levels fall. This drop initiates the shedding of the uterine lining, or menses, to begin again, and a new cycle starts.

Of course, fertilization can't occur without sperm. Created in a man's testes, sperm pass through a series of coiled tubes called the *epididymis,* which stores and nourishes the sperm. The male's contribution to conception then travels through the vas deferens. The prostate gland and seminal vesicles add secretions to the sperm. When a man ejaculates, the sperm mix with fluid to create semen (see Figure 4).

If the sperm are healthy and able to travel, they move from the vagina through the woman's cervix and cervical mucus into the uterine cavity. They can then pass down the fallopian tubes to encounter and hopefully fertilize an egg. It is quite a journey for these sperm, and that is why nature normally provides each man with from 20 million to 100 million sperm to accomplish this task.

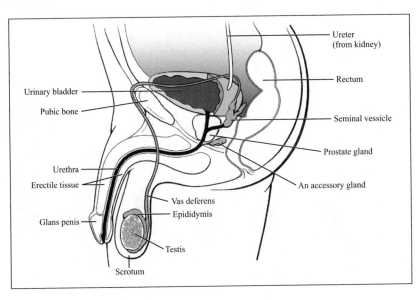

Figure 4: Male reproductive system

Contrary to what some men may like to think, their reproductive abilities are also governed by hormones. Like women, men also use FSH and LH to control their reproductive function. FSH stimulates sperm production, and LH stimulates the production of testosterone.

The Ticking Clock

We may live longer, healthier lives than any previous generation but our reproductive abilities are still on the same clock. As women get older, it is harder for them to conceive. This is because they produce no more eggs than they are born with, and their eggs age as they age. At a certain point, the eggs are no longer fertile.

Fertility rates slide downhill at around age 30 in most women. After 35, the rate of decline is steeper. Once a woman hits 40, her eggs face a challenge analogous to the most difficult black diamond ski run at Vail Mountain. This decline in fertility is all part of the normal aging process and doesn't mean that there is anything wrong with the body (see Figure 5).

Hormones change in women as they age, and menstrual cycles can become shorter or irregular. The chromosomes in female eggs can be dramatically

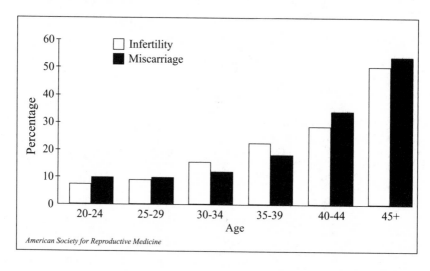

Figure 5: Infertility and miscarriage by age

affected by age. One result might be an irregularity during meiosis. As noted above, just before ovulation, the body creates the LH surge. This stimulates the egg to cut its chromosomes in half from 46 down to 23. If the egg makes a slight mistake and gets rid of 22 chromosomes, it will leave 24 inside the egg. When the sperm enters the egg with its 23 chromosomes, the now fertilized egg will have 47 chromosomes, or one too many.

The presence of this extra chromosome is called *trisomy*. That one extra chromosome can cause lethal problems for the embryo. Often, such embryos will fail to implant, so that pregnancy is thwarted. Even when these embryos do implant, miscarriage is common. It is very unlikely for an embryo with such a defect to lead to a pregnancy. Yet some embryos with trisomy may continue to term. A baby born with Down syndrome has an extra chromosome number 21. This is called trisomy 21. As a woman's age increases, chromosomal abnormalities such as Down syndrome increase. This is why pregnant women in their late thirties and forties are encouraged to have an amniocentesis, which can detect such conditions.

Age can affect the reproductive abilities of men, too, but the effects of age are much less drastic than in women. As men age, their testosterone levels decline and their sexual drive may decrease. The quality of a man's semen also drops as he gets older. There is also evidence that after age 40, a man might have a slightly higher rate of chromosomal abnormalities in his sperm, but this increase is very subtle compared that women's's eggs. On the other hand, most men continue to produce sperm most of their lives. Some have fathered children well into their seventies.

Timing Is Everything

Most people know that timing intercourse is an important part of conception. In fact, there is only a 24- to 48-hour window during the month when conception can occur—that is, just before and just after ovulation. Assuming a woman has a normal 28-day menstrual cycle, ovulation generally occurs around the fourteenth day of the cycle. The window of fertility therefore occurs between approximately cycle day 12 and day 16. Day 1 is best measured as the first day of heavy or full flow.

Once you have charted your cycles and determined how far apart they are, an easy way to approximate when ovulation occurs is to take your cycle lengths and subtract 14. Again, for a 28-day cycle, this would be day 14. For a 32-day cycle, this would be day 18.

This gives you a rough guesstimate as to your ovulation day. Another option is to use a basal body temperature chart. To measure your basal body temperature, you simply take a reading with a special basal body thermometer (a regular thermometer is not sensitive enough) every morning before you start moving around and generating body heat. (Basal thermometers are available at most drug stores.)

You then chart this temperature on a calendar for a month. At the time of ovulation, the temperature should rise or swing up half a degree or more, indicating the time of ovulation. This rise is caused by the production of progesterone around the time of ovulation. It is important to know that the release of the egg—and the time when it is most likely to be fertilized—probably occurs a day before the temperature rise or shift.

A third option for timing ovulation is to use an ovulation predictor kit, available without a prescription at the grocery or drug store. They are relatively easy to use and work by detecting LH in your urine. We advise women to start testing the urine for LH about 4 days prior to their estimated time of ovulation. So, if you predict ovulation is going to be on day 18, start testing your urine around day 14. You should notice no LH surge or color change during the first 2 or 3 days of testing. Then, the day before ovulation, the LH kit should turn positive, suggesting that ovulation will occur in the next 24 to 36 hours, or typically the next day.

Simple Tricks

The following simple tricks may allow you to maximize your chances for conceiving each month on your own without seeking medical care.

○ **LH kits:** Have intercourse 2 days in a row: the night that you have a surge, and the following night.

○ **Temperature charts:** Have intercourse as soon as you notice the temperature rise.

○ **Guesstimating:** Have intercourse 2 days before your estimated ovulation date (which you determine using the cycle length minus 14 days formula), then again on your ovulation date, then again 2 days after.

Fertility Facts

To help you on your quest to become pregnant, let's look at a few facts and clear up some fictions about protecting, preserving, and improving fertility.

Hannah was 30 years old when she met the love of her life. Unfortunately, like many people, she had not given much thought to protecting her fertility earlier in life. When she was in her twenties, Hannah contracted a chlamydia, a sexually transmitted infection, which irreversibly damaged her fallopian tubes. Because of this damage, she had to pursue in vitro fertilization to conceive.

During Hannah's IVF cycle, her ovaries did not respond well because she had been a smoker. Smoking had damaged her eggs and diminished their quality as well. She never imagined that her actions a decade prior would wreak such havoc on her later.

I see patients daily who say "I wish I had known . . . " or, "Why didn't someone tell me . . . ?" The good news is that there are many options available now to correct or bypass problems caused by earlier choices. The bad news is that those treatments can be costly, both financially and emotionally.

Avoiding lifestyle choices that can be detrimental to fertility certainly will not guarantee future pregnancies, but at least in doing so you will avoid any additional complications.

Safe Sex Makes Sense

Sexually transmitted infections (STIs) are a serious threat to male and female fertility. Most STIs can severely limit fertility. Gonorrhea and chlamydia, two very common STIs, can destroy the fallopian tubes. Milder infections also can be detrimental and can even permanently damage the tubes, which is what happened in Hannah's case. More severe infections such as pelvic inflammatory disease (PID) come with a risk of tubal damage of approximately 25 percent per case. Men are vulnerable too. Infections such as gonorrhea and chlamydia can damage sperm passageways and cause scarring that can prevent sperm from developing or significantly decrease the quantity ejaculated.

Other infections, such as human papillomavirus (HPV) can cause precancerous cervical lesions that require surgical procedures such as a loop electrocautery excision procedure (LEEP), freezing of the cervix (cryosurgery), or cold-knife conization to prevent progression to cervical cancer. These surgeries may decrease fertility by altering the cervical mucus. They may also complicate pregnancies later by compromising the cervix, which may lead to preterm labor and delivery or increased risk of cesarean section because of poor dilation.

Other STIs, such as syphilis, hepatitis B and C, and HIV, can threaten your life as well as the lives of your future children. The bottom line is that you should *always* protect yourself from these infections by using barrier method contraception such as a condom. The reality is that there are so many STIs out there that forgetting to use protection even once can affect your life—and your family options—forever. Although condoms are not 100 percent effective, they are the best method to prevent these infections, short of abstinence, of course.

Many of these same infections, such as HIV, hepatitis B and C, and syphilis, can be transmitted nonsexually as well as sexually. Piercings and tattoos are common methods of transmission. If you choose to have these procedures, select a business that uses only new, unopened, sterile instruments. Even one reuse can give you an infection that may never be cured.

Habits That Can Hurt Fertility

Many seemingly simple lifestyle choices can have a big impact on your fertility. Hannah, like many women and men, did herself no favors by smoking cigarettes. Smoking is known to decrease ovarian reserve, which directly affects a woman's ability to have successful pregnancies. This effect is thought to be irreversible.

Smoking cigarettes has been shown to decrease pregnancy rates by nearly 50 percent. In addition, it increases the risk of an ectopic pregnancy (pregnancy in the fallopian tubes). In men, cigarette toxins also cause harm to the sperm and decrease its ability to penetrate eggs. Smoking has no benefits to your health, least of all to your reproductive health. Avoiding smoking throughout your lifetime is simply the wisest plan if you ever hope to have a family, and if you want to live a long and healthy life.

Using illicit substances such as marijuana, cocaine, crack, heroin, and crystal meth poses a serious threat to your fertility. Even if you avoid "heavy" drugs like cocaine, crack, heroin, and crystal meth and use only marijuana, the potential for damage is worse than with legal tobacco products. THC, the active ingredient in marijuana, is a potent inhibitor of the hypothalamic-pituitary axis, the portion of the brain that controls the ovaries and the other glands in the body. Smoking marijuana even occasionally can block ovulation and disrupt the menstrual cycle in women. In men, THC also can decrease sperm production and harm the sperm's ability to penetrate an egg. Again, avoiding these substances is the best way to protect your fertility.

Moderate alcohol consumption is generally not harmful until pregnancy is achieved. For women trying to get pregnant,, I recommend no more than two to four alcoholic drinks per week prior to ovulation. (One drink is equal to a 12-ounce beer, 1 ounce of liquor, or 4 ounces of wine.) Women who hope to become pregnant should abstain completely from alcohol after ovulation. For men, there are less strict regulations regarding alcohol. The general consensus is that men should have no more than five to seven drinks per week, spread out over the week. When a man consumes more alcohol than this, his testosterone levels begin to decrease and estrogen levels begin to increase—a balance that tends to diminish sperm production.

Other Threats to Fertility
Get Fit for Fertility

Men and women don't often realize that weight management is also important for fertility. Overweight or obese people have been shown to have lower rates of fertility. Women who are overweight may not ovulate regularly, and they often have complications during pregnancy. Overweight or obese men have lower sperm counts and generally poorer-quality sperm. Because weight control can be a lifelong struggle that can affect your long-term health as well as your fertility, we recommend controlling your weight before you consider starting a family.

It's also true that you can be too thin for fertility. Low body weight or low body fat also causes problems, especially in women. Low weight due to anorexia, bulimia, or excessive exercise causes ovulatory dysfunction, which is difficult to treat. It also increases pregnancy risks such as preterm labor and delivery. A woman's optimal body mass index (BMI) for conception is between 19 and 25.

Keep It Cool

For men, exposure to heat can be especially problematic for sperm production. The testicles are outside the body for a reason: they produce the best sperm when the testicles are at 95°F rather that the body temperature of 98.6°F. When the testicles are continuously exposed to higher temperatures, sperm production begins to decrease, and the motility of the sperm also starts to suffer. Heat exposure on the job (for example, sitting in a hot seat while operating machinery), or from hot tubs or hot baths, or even from using a laptop, can affect your reproductive abilities.

A few studies have addressed the concern regarding laptop usage and fertility. In men, laptop usage should be confined to a desk or perch off the lap. Whether it is the heat from the laptop, radiation, or some combination of the two, this common device can irreversibly decrease sperm counts.

The medical community increasingly is concerned about the potential threat to fertility caused by cell phones kept near the groin; however, there have not been enough studies done to make a solid judgment on this yet. The best practice to protect your fertility is to keep all electronic devices away from the testicles.

A Male Problem

The brain and the testicles are the two organs in the male body that are protected from the immune system. When there is trauma to the testes, the immune system may be allowed to invade and "see" the sperm—cells that have never been seen before by the body's protection system. When this happens, the body may produce antibodies to the sperm. These antibodies, especially when targeted at the head of the sperm, can act like blinders. Thus, the antibodies can block the sperm from "seeing" or penetrating an egg, even if the egg is right next to it. In rare cases, significant trauma can prevent the testicles from producing sperm. Any trauma, especially if it results in prolonged pain for a day or two, swelling, or bleeding, can cause antisperm antibodies to be produced. The best course of action is to protect the groin from trauma as much as possible, whether it's a fall on the bike seat, a misguided baseball, or a wayward kick in a soccer game. This seems obvious, but we often see male patients who wish they'd been more careful.

Family Matters

Your family history of fertility can give you insight into any potential problems you might face in trying to conceive. A woman should find out whether her mother or grandmothers started menopause early, and whether her mother had multiple miscarriages. Men should find out whether their fathers had problems conceiving children. Both the men and women should find out whether there is a history of mental handicaps or birth defects in their families. Although you can't alter your history, there are ways to prevent problems down the road if you have the facts.

Work Wise

Occupational exposures also can be problematic to fertility. In particular, exposure to radiation or certain chemicals can decrease fertility. For example, a radiology technician or dental hygienist may be exposed to many x-rays at work. It is imperative that those who work with radiation use shield their ovaries and testicles from such exposure. Toluenes, benzenes, and chemotherapeutic agents may also be detrimental to fertility. Using universal precautions to prevent or at least limit these exposures is prudent for people who would like to conceive.

Too Often May Be Too Much

Couples eager to start a family sometimes tell us that they are having sex every day, sometimes for 10 to 20 days in a row. We are all for the joy of sex, but too much of a good thing may actually harm your chances for conception. By the third or fourth consecutive day of intercourse, the male's sperm count actually declines. You don't want to reach the woman's fertile window of opportunity and come up short of enough sperm to achieve a pregnancy. If you are not using a timing method, it is best to have sex every other day to keep up the sperm count.

Fertility Myths

I've heard many myths, falsehoods, and old wives' tales about fertility over the years. Some are just silly; others can put your fertility in jeopardy. Let's look at some common myths and mistakes.

The pill: Many women believe that using birth control pills may decrease their chances of pregnancy later in life. The truth is that the pill is unlikely to affect future fertility at all, either positively or negatively. Nor will the pill delay menopause. A woman who takes the pill for 20 years will not go through menopause 20 years later. Her eggs will still decrease in number while she is on the pill.

Once a woman stops the pill, she will usually return to normal cycles within 1 to 3 months. If she has not started normal periods after 6 months, she should be evaluated to determine why her period hasn't started.

The calendar: There is a popular notion that a couple trying to conceive should have intercourse on menstrual cycle day 14 (where day 1 is the first day of full menstrual flow). However, this practice seems to work for only about 10 percent of women.

The average length of a menstrual cycle is 28 days; however, the normal range is 24 to 35 days. For a woman who has a 35-day cycle, intercourse on day 14 would most likely be far too early to result in pregnancy. To calculate the day she is most likely to be fertile, a woman should subtract 14 from the cycle length. For example, a woman with a 35-day cycle should be fertile on day 21. However, this is just an average, and the window of fertility may vary quite a bit during the cycle.

The charts: When "tracking" their fertility, many couples start with the basal body temperature method. It is easy, cheap, and fairly effective. Basal body temperature increases about 0.5 to 1 degree after ovulation.

However, many women who use this method try to time intercourse on the day the temperature rises. But this rise in temperature occurs 1 to 3 days *after* ovulation occurs, and this is not an effective time. Multiple studies have shown that conception increases when intercourse occurs *before* the egg is released, not afterward, as couples often believe with temperature charting.

There is a similar misunderstanding about tracking mucus changes—when the cervical mucus changes to a clear consistency like egg whites, ovulation has already occurred.

The kits: Ovulation predictor kits are readily available over the counter at most pharmacies. They come in many varieties: some with two lines, some with smiley faces, and some digital. They all assess for the same hormone—luteinizing hormone (LH), which triggers ovulation. The test strips are used in the morning, and when the kits test positive, ovulation will usually occur in the next 24 to 36 hours. Couples sometimes assume they should have sex as many times as possible at this point. Although doing so will serve the purpose, it is probably a bit much. Optimal timing for intercourse is the day that the kit tests positive and the day afterward. What you do the rest of the month is entirely up to you and your partner. But we wish you good luck!

The diets: There also are many misconceptions about supplements and foods and whether they enhance fertility. A specific diet plan, whether it involves eating a lot of pineapples, ice cream, or gluten-free foods, will not likely enhance your fertility. When counseling patients about diet, I recommend a healthy, well-balanced diet that doesn't venture to any extremes. Still, even that doesn't likely enhance fertility, but it does promote better health in general.

The stress: We receive many inquiries about the impact of stress on fertility, because women who want to start a family do get anxious when they can't get pregnant right away. Women face stress in their regular, daily lives, so it is impossible to remove that aspect completely. What effect does it have on fertility? The answer is difficult to quantify. Certain known stressors, such as the death of a parent, a job change, relocation, and divorce, have a definite effect on pregnancy rates.

But what about the day-to-day pressures of work and home life? The effects of this kind of stress are less definite. Our advice is to decrease stress as much as possible, using methods such as massage, yoga, exercise, fun with friends and family, and that proven remedy, a good night's sleep. A reduction in stress may not improve your chances of becoming pregnant, but it will help you to cope with the challenges involved in fighting for your fertility.

Adoption Cure

Nancy and Greg had been married for more than 10 years, and they'd been trying to start a family for at least 8 years. They had tried the fertility drug Clomid (clomiphene citrate) as well as intrauterine insemination, surgery, and finally IVF, five times. Finally, they decided to pursue adoption. After 2 years, they received a call that an adoptable child was waiting for them—finally, they'd have a family. After enjoying their adopted daughter, Laura, for just 3 months, Nancy began to notice breast tenderness and morning sickness. She was 2 months pregnant! How could this have happened, after all they had been through?

We hear similar stories all the time about couples giving up on fertility treatments, adopting, and then getting pregnant. As research has demonstrated, adoption is not a good way to get pregnant. Though it makes sense that the stress of infertility is over when you adopt, there is no research showing that it improves pregnancy. More than likely, the right egg met the right sperm at just the right time, and one of life's great miracles occurred.

Subsequent Pregnancies

We also often hear people say that women who conceived easily with their first baby will conceive the second one even more easily. Unfortunately, this is not always the case. Amanda, 33, and her husband, Corey, decided they were ready to start a family. She stopped the birth control pill and became pregnant 1 month later. She enjoyed her pregnancy and gave birth to a son, Gage. After a year, they were ready to begin trying to have a second baby. Three years later, it still had not happened.

Many couples believe that because they've had one successful pregnancy, they will never have to face infertility. However, it's not unheard of for couples to face challenges with a second pregnancy.

When to Seek Help

If you and your partner have a healthy lifestyle and you have been following generally prescribed methods for timing your intercourse but still have not been able to become pregnant and sustain the pregnancy, don't wait too long to see a fertility specialist. Many couples who don't have successful pregnancies in their first attempts simply keep trying, hoping that next month will be "the month."

Fertility experts usually recommend that when a woman under the age of 35 has been trying to conceive for at least 1 year without success, she should begin a fertility evaluation to determine whether there are physical or medical challenges thwarting her efforts.

Studies show that a couple's ability to get pregnant drops the longer they try to achieve pregnancy. And the older the woman is, the harder it gets.

A woman older than 35 should probably see a fertility specialist if she's been trying to get pregnant for 6 months. Couples who are aware of potential problems such as a low sperm count, a history of pelvic infections, gynecologic surgeries, irregular menstrual cycles, or more than two miscarriages should not put off a fertility evaluation any longer than a month or two.

Now that you understand how the basic physiology of the female and male reproductive systems works, and how fertility can be affected by lifestyle and habits, we will move on in the next chapter and look at the major medical causes of infertility. Once we have a clear understanding of what a patient's particular problem or diagnosis is, the treatments become easier. Remember, with all of the innovations available to infertility patients today, nearly everyone has a chance to have a baby.

Chapter Two

Become Your Own Best Advocate

THE FIRST STEP in fighting infertility is to identify the best doctor and clinic for you—one that will perform the thorough evaluation you need to determine your specific fertility challenges. Very few obstetrician-gynecologists invest significant time and effort in understanding infertility in all of its forms. Only those who have made it a major part of their medical practices will do a thorough job with basic evaluation.

For most sophisticated procedures, I advise you to see an infertility specialist—not someone who delivers babies or performs general gynecologic surgery. Obviously, I have a bias in this regard because I am an infertility specialist. While OB-GYNs are essential to maintaining your reproductive health and (hopefully) delivering your baby, they are mostly focused on surgery and obstetrics. Fertility specialists, on the other hand, can offer the full scope of tests and treatments that you might require. Too many women and men want to be "good patients." They trust that their regular gynecologists or obstetricians are well trained and up-to-date in fertility treatments. This is like assuming that your computer technician can fix an airplane engine, too. Rarely can someone be a master of more than one area in such a complex, ever-changing medical field.

Whether you rely on your OB-GYN or a fertility specialist, I encourage you to educate yourself and to serve as your own advocate by asking informed questions. I cannot tell you how many times frantic and frustrated patients have come to our clinic after spending months, even years, undergoing treatments that were prescribed without clear diagnoses.

Selecting a Doctor and Clinic

When you are looking for a fertility specialist, you might start by checking with friends or coworkers who have been through successful treatments. You might also seek the advice of your general practitioner or your OB-GYN and other contacts in the medical community.

I strongly recommend, however, that you rely primarily on your own research based on your specific needs and situation. To evaluate a particular fertility clinic or reproductive center by its track record, you can visit the Web sites for the Centers for Disease Control and Prevention (www.cdc.gov), or the Society of Assisted Reproductive Technologies (SART, www.sart.org), which is associated with the American Society for Reproductive Medicine (ASRM). These sites provide the success rates of all SART members in the United States with regard to in vitro fertilization and egg donation. The CDC collects and audits this data and allows patients to view the relative success rates of different centers and clinics. Also, the American Society for Reproductive Medicine or ASRM (www.asrm.org), and RESOLVE: The National Infertility Association (www.resolve.org) offer physician referral resources on their Web sites.

While you may not need in vitro fertilization—at least initially—clinics that perform this sophisticated procedure with high success rates generally have the staff and expertise necessary to perform basic infertility testing and less aggressive treatments as well. Still, there are only a handful of IVF clinics that have consistent high levels of success, advanced labs, and proven diagnostic skills, so you need to be a discriminating patient.

It is tempting for many patients to choose a fertility clinic based on location, but keep in mind you are not going for groceries—you are fighting for your dream of having a family. This can be a very expensive battle, so while it might seem practical to minimize your travel costs, you will only waste resources if you choose the wrong facility. You should make your decision based on which clinic or physician has the best track record in dealing with your particular fertility challenge.

ASRM has offered the following guidelines to use when you are selecting a fertility clinic:

○ The qualifications and experience of physicians and staff

○ The types of patients each clinic treats

○ The support services they offer

○ The clinic's fees compared with others'

○ The clinic's record on live birth rates and multiple pregnancy rates

Note that older clinics' birth rates are based on years of experience. Small and new programs may still be well qualified, even though they may still be determining their success rates.

Every couple wants to use the most successful clinic, but many factors contribute to the overall success of a program. You should not choose your clinic solely on its published pregnancy rates. Some clinics may be willing to accept patients with a low chance of live birth, while others do not, which means their pregnancy success rates aren't comparable. A clinic may specialize in certain types of infertility treatments that either help or hinder its success in producing live births.

Credibility is important, too. Here is a checklist of questions to consider in determining which clinic you choose.

○ Does the program adhere to the guidelines set forth by the ASRM?

○ Is the program a member of the Society of Assisted Reproductive Technologies (SART)?

○ Is the IVF lab accredited by the College of American Pathologists or by the Joint Commission? (These organizations require assisted reproductive technology programs to have staff members trained in reproductive endocrinology, laparoscopic surgery, sonography, hormone measurement, tissue culture technique, and sperm/egg interaction.)

○ Does the program report its results to SART and CDC? (The compiled results are published in *Fertility and Sterility*, the ASRM journal, and are available on the Web sites for SART and the CDC.)

○ How many physicians will be involved in my care?

○ To what degree will my own physician participate in my care?

○ What types of counseling and support services are available?

○ Is there someone in the program whom I can call day or night if I have a problem?

- Does the facility freeze embryos (cryopreservation)?

- Are donor sperm available in the program? Donor eggs? Donor embryos?

- Does the program have a cutoff for age or basal FSH (follicle-stimulating hormone) levels?

- Based on my medical history, how many embryos are likely to be transferred to my uterus? (Transferring too many embryos would unnecessarily increase your risk for multiple births.)

- Who makes the final decision to cancel treatment if my response is less than optimal?

Measuring the Success of a Clinic or Program

If a clinic or program cites a birth rate for each procedure it offers, be sure that the program representative counts twins as one successful pregnancy, not two. When you discuss recent assisted reproduction performance with a clinic, keep in mind that the birth rate may vary depending on the denominator used—for example, per cycle started, per retrieval, or per embryo transfer. The rate per cycle refers to the number of pregnancies per the number of patients who start on a cycle of fertility drugs, even if they don't have an egg retrieval. The rate per retrieval means the number of pregnancies among all patients who make it to the stage of having their eggs retrieved. The rate per transfer means the number of pregnancies among all patients who make it to the stage of having embryos to put back in the uterus.

For example, birth rates per egg retrieval do not include cancelled fertility drug cycles, and rates per embryo transfer do not include cancelled cycles or eggs that were retrieved but failed to become fertilized. Therefore, birth rates per cycle are higher per egg retrieval and are highest per embryo transfer.

Your First Appointment

Make no mistake; dealing with infertility is usually a very emotional experience. Yet I would not advise you to settle on a clinic or a physician based on your personal compatibility or relationships with a physician or a clinic's staff members. The skill levels of the doctor and nurses and the quality of the work done by the IVF laboratory team are the most important factors.

Once you have selected a clinic or center based on its ability to help you have a child, then you can begin your search within it to find individual staff members whom you trust and feel comfortable with. Once you have chosen a physician, your clinic will schedule an initial consultation. Let's look at what you should know going into this first appointment.

You probably will be asked to fill out a health questionnaire before that first visit, to describe your medical history. On the day of your consultation, you may be asked to bring your medical records, particularly those relating to your reproductive health. This includes the woman's gynecological records and the male's urological records. This first meeting might include a tour of the clinic, introductions to key staff, and time with your physician.

This is the physician's opportunity to evaluate and interview you and your partner. The doctor needs to know the regularity of your menstrual cycles. There will also be questions about whether you have had any abnormal bleeding or pelvic pain, whether you have any history of pelvic infection, whether you have used an IUD for birth control, and whether you have had abnormal Pap smears. You should also tell the physician about any surgeries you've had related to your gynecologic organs.

The doctor also will want to know the male partner's history, including any pregnancies he has been involved with, any sperm testing he has undergone, and any urological health complications he has had. Make note of any medications you and your partner are taking, and whether you drink alcohol, use tobacco, or drink caffeine. It is also important to tell your doctor about any environmental exposures you might be subjected to, either through your lifestyle or your employment.

An experienced infertility specialist may well get a good fix on the source of a couple's infertility problem just from this initial consultation. Among the most obvious tip-offs:

O Women who have menstrual cycles only two to three times per year are typically not ovulating. At the very least, they will require medications to cause a resumption of their ovulatory cycles on a monthly basis.

○ Males with a history of undescended testicles or low sperm count are often infertile.

Your physician may perform a physical exam during this initial visit to see if there are anatomic clues to your problem. A woman might also be asked to take an initial pelvic ultrasound to get an image of your reproductive organs. This ultrasound helps your physician determine whether you have uterine fibroids, ovarian cystic structures that would suggest endometriosis, or a dilated, fluid-filled fallopian tube, which would suggests tubal blockage.

If the cause of your infertility is not obvious at this stage, a basic infertility workup or evaluation will be in order. You want a thorough evaluation, which can take three or four office visits to complete. This is a troubleshooting procedure that looks at your reproductive processes to find out what is keeping you from having a successful pregnancy.

To help you understand the workup, let's go through the evaluation process step by step, following the stages of conception.

Step One

For a woman to conceive, the male's sperm must arrive at her cervix. So, one of the steps is to do a sperm analysis on the male. He will be asked to abstain from sexual activity for 2 to 7 days. Then a sperm sample will be collected either at the clinic or at home. If it is collected at home, it will need to be collected in a container from the clinic and delivered within 30 to 35 minutes of collection. The initial parameters evaluated during this test will include:

○ The volume of semen, the liquid that the sperm reside in

○ The total number of sperm present in the sample

○ The number of sperm per milliliter of semen, known as the sperm concentration, or count

○ The *motility* of the sperm (that is, the percentage of sperm that are swimming or moving)

○ The shape of the sperm

○ The presence of white blood cells (a sign of infection in the reproductive tract)

CHARACTERISTICS OF NORMAL SPERM

Count	> 20 million per mL
Motility	> 40% of sperm
Morphology	> 4% by strict criteria (*varies by laboratory*)
Culture	Negative for infection
Antisperm Antibody	Negative

Often the semen is sent for a culture to further evaluate for infection. Some men may also be tested for what are called *antisperm antibodies*. Antibodies are usually made by the immune system against foreign invaders such as bacteria or viruses. Sometimes the body gets tricked into making antibodies against itself. In this case of antisperm antibodies, men's bodies produce antibodies against the sperm, rendering the sperm unable to fertilize an egg. Unless there is a specialized antisperm antibody test, this problem will be missed in the routine semen analysis. Men who have had testicular infection, trauma, or surgery on their reproductive organs are particularly at risk for the presence of antibodies.

Step Two

Next, the sperm must move through the cervix into the uterine cavity. To make certain this is possible, your physician will perform a postcoital examination to test the cervical mucus. Female bodies produce watery cervical mucus that allows the sperm to swim from the vagina up into the uterus, but only for 2 to 3 days per month—those days immediately before ovulation. So, this test must be timed to occur 1 to 2 days prior to ovulation, on day 12 or 13 of the menstrual cycle.

You will be asked to have intercourse either the night before the test or the morning of the test. The procedure will be similar to a Pap smear. During a pelvic exam, the cervical mucus is aspirated from the cervix. By examining this mucus under a microscope, the physician can determine if sperm are present and alive, swimming purposefully through the mucus on their way to the uterine cavity.

For some women there is a lack of mucus entirely. This suggests a problem with the glands of the cervix and their ability to make mucus. In other cases the mucus may be very thick, or viscous, so that it impedes the sperm. The physician also might find that the mucus appears entirely normal, but there are no sperm present.

Step Three

Then, the sperm must be able to swim through the uterine cavity and out to the distal part of the fallopian tubes, where fertilization occurs, to reach the egg. Once it is determined that sperm can enter the uterine cavity, your physician will look to see that the uterine cavity itself is normal and that the fallopian tubes are open. The standard test used to evaluate the uterus and tubes together is known as the *hysterosalpingogram,* or (thankfully) the HSG.

This examination is done typically between cycle days 5 and 10 and involves an x-ray. This procedure also begins like a typical pelvic exam. A speculum is inserted, then a small catheter is placed through the cervix and into the lower part of the uterine cavity. Through this small catheter, fluid is injected that shows up as a contrast on the x-ray film.

After this fluid is injected into the uterus, the uterine cavity fills and is outlined so that your physician can detect defects such as polyps, fibroids, or an abnormal shape to the uterine cavity. The fluid then travels down the fallopian tubes and hopefully spills out the ends. X-ray films are taken of this fluid filling and spilling from the ends of the tubes so your doctor can detect any tubal blockage.

Mild menstrual cramping typically occurs with an HSG and can be lessened by taking ibuprofen one hour prior to the exam. Patients who are especially sensitive to uterine manipulations or cramping may benefit from Valium before the exam. It is important to begin taking antibiotics on the day of the exam and to continue them for at least 4 days to minimize the risks of infection. You should not undergo this examination if you are allergic to iodine, because the fluid used to image the uterus and tubes contains an iodine-like substance. Only a very low level of radiation is released during the HSG, so it poses no risk to fertility. The HSG should not be done if there's a chance you may be pregnant.

Step Four

By this point, your physician has done tests to establish whether:

1. The male's sperm is able to fertilize an egg,

2. His sperm can travel through cervical mucus, and

3. The sperm can get into the uterine cavity and down the fallopian tubes where an egg should be waiting.

The fourth test is done to determine if an egg is available and waiting for the sperm to fertilize it, or in other words, to determine whether ovulation is occurring.

One of the best ways to determine if ovulation is occurring is to actually view the process with vaginal ultrasound. This allows your physician to see whether the follicle (the sac of fluid containing the egg) is growing and enlarging in the few days before ovulation. Immediately after ovulation, the vaginal ultrasound also allows the doctor to see whether the follicle has ruptured or collapsed to released the egg and fluid from the follicle into the abdominal cavity.

Twenty-four to 36 hours before ovulation, the pituitary gland in the brain releases luteinizing hormone (LH), as we saw in Chapter 1. This triggers the rupture of the follicle and the release of the egg. Many urine-based kits, which are sold over-the-counter at grocery stores and pharmacies, allow patients to detect this so-called LH surge approximately 1 day before ovulation, and this is also an important test that doctors perform. The LH surge suggests—but does not totally prove—that ovulation is occurring.

Your doctor might also test for the presence of progesterone, which is produced by the ovaries only if ovulation occurs. The test is typically performed 7 to 8 days after ovulation—around day 21 of a 28-day menstrual cycle—when your doctor will draw blood to obtain a blood progesterone measurement. A level greater than 10 nanograms indicates that ovulation is taking place.

Additional Tests for the First Round

Checking Your Eggs

Among the questions that might remain at this point in a patient's first workup are those concerning the quality of the female's eggs. Interestingly, all women seem to have eggs that are genetically programmed to last a certain number of years, but that number varies from woman to woman. Some 30-year-old women may have eggs that have aged prematurely and are virtually near menopause. Other women may be in their mid-forties and have eggs that are still viable.

Fortunately, there are simple tests to assess the quality and relative age of each woman's eggs. One of the earliest tests for egg quality is the measurement of follicle stimulating hormone, or FSH. This hormone carries the brain's signal to the eggs during the menstrual cycle. The louder the brain must talk with FSH to get the attention of the eggs, the lower the quality of those eggs.

If the FSH level is low, indicating that the brain is simply "whispering" to the eggs and triggering ovulation, the eggs are in good shape. If an FSH level is high, showing that the brain is yelling and screaming just to get one egg out a month, there is a bit of a problem.

This blood test is typically done on the second or third day of the menstrual cycle. An FSH level of less than 10 international units is considered normal in most laboratories. However, there are a few caveats of FSH measurement. The reason the test should be done on day 2 or 3 of the menstrual cycle is that, on this day, a woman's estrogen levels should be under 50; but if the estrogen level is above 50, it will suppress FSH and make it look falsely normal. If this occurs, the test must be repeated the following month.

Clinics and centers may use different machines to measure FSH, so the methodologies can vary quite a bit from clinic to clinic. It is important to know the range of normal in the clinic where you are being tested. Ask them at what FSH level they see problems with a woman's fertility.

The Clomid Challenge Test

The clomiphene citrate challenge test (CCCT, or Clomid challenge test) is a modified version of the FSH test that some clinics may use. It involves measuring FSH on day 2 or 3, but in addition, the woman takes 100 milligrams of Clomid (clomiphene citrate) on cycle days 5 through 9, and then her physician measures FSH levels on day 10. Clomid is designed to stimulate the ovary to release more eggs by making the pituitary increase FSH levels, which spurs follicle growth. If this process is successful, a healthy, egg-bearing follicle—or several of them—should be present by day 10.

Healthy follicles produce a hormone called *inhibin*, which feeds back to the pituitary gland and shuts down or blocks FSH production. Therefore, by day 10, if the Clomid has recruited healthy eggs, FSH levels should be low. If FSH levels are high on day 10, it suggests that a healthy follicle did not result from stimulating the ovary and that inhibin production did not occur. If FSH is above 10 on either day 3 or day 10 of a Clomid challenge test, it is considered abnormal. Elevated FSH indicates poor egg quality and therefore suggests a poor prognosis for a natural pregnancy.

Egg Ultrasound

Another way that your physician may assess the function and health of the eggs in your ovaries is to look at each ovary on an ultrasound. Although one egg grows in a follicle each month and ultimately ovulates, there are many other eggs waiting their turn in small follicles called *antral follicles*. These small sacs of fluid are lined by cells called *granulosa cells*, and each contains an egg. On the ultrasound, your doctor can see the number of follicles present in the ovary.

The more eggs each ovary contains, the healthier that ovary is, and, typically, the healthier the eggs are. Conversely, your doctor can also see whether an ovary is shrinking and contains only one or two follicles.

Anti-Mullerian Hormone Testing

There is also a promising new test for egg quality that looks at levels of a hormone called *anti-mullerian hormone* (AMH), which is released by the granulosa cells lining each follicle. The more eggs a woman has waiting in the wings to grow, the more AMH they will be making, suggesting that there are more and better eggs available for conception. Once your doctor has looked at your FSH, your antral follicle counts, your AMH levels, and possibly even your Clomid challenge test, he or she should know if your eggs have the potential to produce a healthy embryo and, therefore, whether you can conceive a child.

The only major questions remaining at this point in your initial round of fertility tests are:

○ Can the egg released from the ovary actually travel into the fallopian tube or get picked up by the fallopian tube?

○ Can the egg get fertilized?

Whether an egg can travel from the ovary to the tube can be a difficult question to answer. Typical impediments to this process are adhesions within the tube, or a condition known as endometriosis. Unfortunately, neither of these conditions can be diagnosed with simple office tests. They require a minor surgery under general anesthesia. The surgery, known as laparoscopy, detects the presence of adhesions or scar tissue. Laparoscopy involves inserting a small telescope through the belly button to get a view of the uterus, fallopian tubes, ovaries, and the entire peritoneal cavity. It gives your doctor far more information than HSG, which only confirms that the tubes are open.

While it is effective at diagnosing adhesions and endometriosis, the laparoscopy is clearly more invasive than any of the other tests discussed so far. It is also more expensive. Often, therefore, physicians do not suggest that patients undergo laparoscopy if the other basic tests already have revealed a specific problem.

Egg Fertilization Tests

Physicians also face a challenge in assessing whether your eggs are actually being fertilized. Presumptive evidence of fertilization can be obtained by testing the sperm. However, even semen that tests as normal sometimes fails to penetrate or fertilize eggs. The only absolute way to know whether the sperm is doing its job correctly is to perform in vitro fertilization. This entails combining the sperm with the eggs in a petri dish and observing the occurrence of fertilization over a 16-hour period. Unfortunately, this is not practical as a test and is rarely pursued unless other information suggests the couple needs in vitro fertilization.

After the First Round of Tests

Once the basic tests have been performed (see "Female Fertility Tests," on this page), your physician usually has identified a specific factor causing your infertility. At this point, you will meet with your doctor and go over all test results. If a specific problem is identified—for example, if the cervical mucus is the only problem revealed during the workup—your doctor will recommend a treatment plan.

In the case of poor cervical mucus, for example, the physician would probably recommend that their team "wash" your husband's sperm and inject it into the uterus, a process known as intrauterine insemination. This "airlifts" or carries your husband's sperm past the cervix and into the uterus directly, bypassing the mucus.

Other possible diagnosis and treatment plans include:

○ Ovulation disorders, which are usually treated with fertility medications

○ Low sperm count, which is treated with insemination, though a urologist may be asked to determine if there is an organic cause for the male's low sperm production

○ Uterine cavity or fallopian tube problems, which are usually addressed surgically

FEMALE FERTILITY TESTS

○ Post-coital test

○ Hysterosalpingogram (HSG)

○ Baseline ultrasound

○ Ultrasound documenting follicular rupture (ovulation)

○ Luteal phase prograsterone

○ Thyroid panel

○ Hormones (estradiol, follicle-stimulating hormone, anti-mullerian hormone)

○ Blood type

○ Rubella

○ Varicella

The good news is that no matter what the problem is, there is usually a treatment available. You can discuss your treatment plans with your physician once the test results have been analyzed from your initial workup. That is when you learn what the treatment will be, how much it will cost, what the success rate of the treatment is, and the logistical steps for that course of treatment.

Recommended Additional Tests

During the initial evaluation, I generally recommend some additional tests that aren't directly related to infertility. These are tests designed to ensure the optimum health of your baby should conception occur. I like to check a woman's blood type, because if her blood type is Rh negative it makes pregnancy a bit more complicated and requires specific medications such as RhoGAM for any bleeding during pregnancy. I also check for antibodies or immunity to both German measles, or rubella, and chicken pox, or varicella. If any of these viruses occurs in the first trimester, they can cause major fetal anomalies. Therefore, if a patient is not immune, she should be vaccinated before beginning fertility treatments.

There are also genetic tests that we offer to couples planning a family. One screens for cystic fibrosis, a single-gene disorder that causes both lung and gastrointestinal problems in the offspring. This gene can be tested for in the parents' blood to determine if they are carriers and at risk of passing it on to their offspring. There are other genetic disorders that are prevalent in certain ethnic groups, such as African Americans, the Jewish population, French Canadians, and Southeast Asians.

Talk to your physician or a genetic counselor if you are interested in genetic tests. Chapter 16 has more in-depth information on genetic testing.

During the initial workup period at my clinic, I talk with my patients about certain lifestyle precautions they can take to optimize their pregnancies. I prescribe prenatal vitamins for all women who plan to conceive, because nutrition is important for optimal health. It is also true that the folic acid present in prenatal vitamins can lower the risk of having a baby with spinal cord defects.

I advise patients that they should not lose or gain weight rapidly, as both can throw off ovulation. Before conceiving, being at near-normal body weight is certainly optimal. Being overweight during pregnancy can increase the risk of pregnancy complications such as hypertension and gestational diabetes. Physical exercise at moderate levels can help maintain normal body weight while reducing stress. Continuing moderate exercise into pregnancy has also been shown to be beneficial.

The initial infertility workup may seem daunting at first, but most couples find that taking positive steps to deal with their infertility concerns gives them not only relief from their worries, but hope, too. As you go through the tests and, step by step, eliminate or deal with problems, you begin to feel that you are back in control and on the path toward your dream of starting a family.

CHAPTER THREE

Treatment Strategies for Your Fertility Challenge

TABITHA CAME TO us after struggling for three years to conceive. A quick check of her medical history revealed, to my surprise, that her obstetrician-gynecologist had not done any testing before putting Tabitha on Clomid (clomiphene citrate), a common medication for infertile women with ovulation disorders. It is designed to stimulate the ovaries to grow more eggs. Unfortunately, Clomid is often overprescribed for patients challenged by infertility. I've often thought about taking out ads in national magazines and newspapers to caution people that fertility pills are not always the answer to their problems. Fertility pills are not cure-alls. In fact, they are very limited in their effectiveness.

For 18 months, Tabitha, took the drug, which was a waste of time and money and did not result in pregnancy. When we tested her and Tim, her husband, it became clear that Tabitha was fine. There was nothing wrong with her reproductive system. Tim, however, had a very low sperm count.

I told this frustrated couple the bad news first: The drug she'd been taking was not right in her case. Then I gave her the good news: She could likely become pregnant if we used a procedure we have refined at our clinic. We would inject Tim's sperm into her eggs to overcome their infertility.

I'm happy to report that Tim and Tabitha eventually had a healthy child.

Still, this couple could have been parents nearly three years earlier if they'd gone to a physician who did the proper array of tests on both of them.

Infertility patients are vulnerable. They desperately want a baby. Often, their emotions overwhelm them to the point that they fail to ask questions and demand answers of their physicians.

To arm you with the ability to choose appropriate infertility therapy, this chapter provides you with general descriptions of the most successful treatments, drugs, and procedures used by well-trained physicians who specialize in the latest infertility treatments. I will go deeper into specific treatments in later chapters.

Three Strategies
for Treating Infertility

It's helpful to think of fertility treatment as falling into three categories. The first is *ovulation induction*.

Ovulation induction is a method for helping a woman when she is having difficulty ovulating—releasing the normal one egg each month. It is also a procedure for helping a woman make extra eggs each month. By making extra eggs, you "expand the field," so to speak, for the sperm. If a sperm has more than one egg to fertilize, then the chances are higher for pregnancy.

A second category of fertility treatments is artificial insemination, also known as *intrauterine insemination* (IUI). The decidedly non-medical term for this is the "turkey-baster method." By whatever name, this is a process in which sperm are washed and concentrated and placed at the top of the uterus so more sperm reach the egg or eggs. Again the goal is to increase the chances for fertilization and pregnancy.

The third category we'll look at is *in vitro fertilization* (IVF). In this method of fertility treatment a women takes medication to markedly increase the number of eggs that she makes in a month. Then the eggs are extracted and fertilized *outside* her body. The fertilized eggs are then grown in a lab culture for 3 or 5 days. Then they are placed directly into her uterine cavity.

Now let's look at each of these three treatment methods in more detail.

Ovulation Induction

Ovulation induction can be accomplished with either oral or injectable medications. The most commonly prescribed oral medication is one I've already mentioned a couple times—clomiphene citrate, also known by the trademarked brand names Clomid and Serophene. This is a perfectly good drug as long as it is used properly and prescribed for patients whom it can help. This medication is typically taken for 5 days over a month starting either on day 3 or 5 of a woman's cycle.

We recommend a pelvic exam prior to starting Clomid to make certain that you do not have any cysts on your ovaries, as Clomid can cause those cysts to grow. Clomid is an estrogen receptor blocker, which means it prevents your body from responding to estrogen. Clomid essentially tricks your body into thinking it is menopausal, so your pituitary gland compensates by increasing follicle-stimulating hormone (FSH) and luteinizing hormone (LH). The increased FSH and LH stimulate the ovaries to make an extra egg.

About 20 percent of women taking Clomid report side effects. The most common are hot flashes, mood swings, and headaches. An extremely rare side effect reported with Clomid is visual changes—either bright spots or afterimages, where you look at something and then look away, yet still see that initial image. If you have any visual changes, it is important that you stop the Clomid and call your doctor.

Clomid can induce egg development in about 80 percent of women who are not ovulating. Pregnancy rates, however, are much lower and depend on many factors, such as a woman's age, the state of her fallopian tubes, and her partner's sperm health.

It is true for almost all fertility treatments that the younger a woman is, the greater the likelihood that treatment will be successful.

○ For women 37 years old or younger, the success rate for Clomid is approximately 8 to 10 percent per month.

○ For those 38 to 40 years old the success rate is 6 to 7 percent per month.

○ For those 41 to 42 years old, the success rate is 3 to 4 percent per month.

○ For those above 42 years, the success rate is less than 1 percent per month.

Those statistics assume that a woman has two open fallopian tubes and her partner's sperm parameters are within normal range. If a woman has only one functional tube, the success rates would be about half the above rates.

Too often women come to us after their doctors have had them take Clomid for many months—even years—without becoming pregnant. Usually we find they have been given the wrong treatment for their particular problems. In these cases, the patients are highly frustrated.

The vast majority of Clomid-induced pregnancies will occur within the first 4 to 6 months of taking it, so there is little benefit from continuing Clomid much beyond this time frame. Most clinicians will limit Clomid prescriptions to no more than 6 months. No one knows why the success rate drops after these first few months—but there are a couple of possible reasons.

Because it is an estrogen receptor blocker, Clomid can reduce the quantity and wateriness of cervical mucus, which presents a barrier for sperm. Intra-uterine insemination can overcome this side effect by placing the sperm past the cervix and into the uterus. Clomid can also alter the endometrium, making it thin and unreceptive to implantation. These issues with the cervical mucus and uterine lining may explain why success rates decrease with prolonged use of Clomid.

There are many ways that you can assess whether you are ovulating with Clomid. Most doctors rely on the menstrual pattern, ovulation prediction kits, measurement of serum progesterone levels, or the basal body temperature chart to monitor a patient's response to the standard dose of Clomid.

If there is still doubt about whether you are ovulating, your caregiver may examine the ovaries with ultrasound to determine if and when ovulation took place. With ultrasound, the follicle containing the egg can be watched as it progressively grows and then disappears, confirming the release of the egg. If ovulation does not occur at the usual 50-milligram dosage, Clomid may be increased by 50-milligram increments in subsequent cycles until ovulation is achieved.

Although dosages in excess of 100 milligrams are not approved by the Food and Drug Administration, your physician may elect to increase the dose to 150 or 200 milligrams. Occasionally, the physician may choose to add other medications if Clomid alone is not inducing ovulation.

Women who cannot tolerate the medication or those with a pituitary tumor should not use Clomid or any form of clomiphene citrate. Additionally, Clomid is very unlikely to work if the male's sperm counts are below a certain threshold level, if there is tubal blockage, or if there is a pituitary cause for infertility.

There are other oral medications used for ovulation induction. Some belong to a group called *aromatase inhibitors*. Aromatase inhibitors are medications that reduce estrogen levels. Although these medications are currently FDA-approved for postmenopausal breast cancer, two drugs—letrozole (Femara) and anastrozole (Arimidex)—have been used successfully for ovulation induction.

Typically, these pills are prescribed for 5 days starting on cycle day 3, 4, or 5. Studies indicate that pregnancy rates are comparable to those with Clomid. These medications tend to create fewer side effects than Clomid, yet they have not been used for fertility treatment for as long as Clomid has, so the safety profile is not as well established. Letrozole seems to work similar to Clomid in treating ovulation disorders; however, there has been a study suggesting that babies born after letrozole treatment have more birth defects. Therefore, most doctors are sticking with Clomid.

Tamoxifen (sold under the brand name Soltamox) is another oral medication shown to induce ovulation in women. Tamoxifen is another estrogen receptor blocker. You may have heard of its being used to treat breast cancer.

Keep in mind that the more eggs you produce each month, the greater the likelihood you will have more than one baby. With oral medications, the twin rate is approximately 7 to 8 percent. Three or more babies per pregnancy are very rare—less than 1 percent—but possible!

The other group of medications used for ovulation induction are broadly referred to as *gonadotropins*. These are injectable medications that are mostly synthetic forms of FSH or FSH and LH. These are the same hormones that an ovulatory woman makes on her own every month, but in higher concentrations that help produce more than one egg each month.

Gonadotropins are much more effective at producing multiple eggs than Clomid is; hence the need to be monitored much more closely with these medications. If your body makes eight eggs in response to these medications and all eight fertilize, you could have a much larger family than desired.

I am fairly certain you have no interest in a large, instant family, so it is important for your physician to monitor you closely while taking these medications. Monitoring is done with blood tests for estradiol levels and vaginal sonograms to detect how many eggs are developing and when they are "ready."

The eggs are considered mature when the follicle (the fluid-filled cyst they grow in) measures 15 to 18 millimeters in average diameter. During a typical month of gonadotropin administration, it is likely that you will be scheduled for three to six visits. The goal is to produce from two to four mature eggs.

When the appropriate number of eggs reach just the right size, a second medication is usually given. This is called a "trigger shot," which is not as scary as it sounds. This type of "trigger shot" causes your eggs to ovulate at a specific time so that you can make certain the sperm are on board at the right time—often through insemination, which will be discussed later.

The gonadotropins go by several names. The common trade names are Follistim, Gonal-F, Repronex, and Menopur. For the trigger shot, either Ovidrel, gonadotropin, or a *gonadotropin-releasing hormone agonist*—a synthetic peptide that prompts the release of FSH and LH—can be used. These medications are

A TYPICAL CLOMID TREATMENT CYCLE

You will quickly discover that infertility treatment has its own vocabulary. "Starting a cycle" is one of the more common terms. The following is a step-by-step treatment cycle for patients using Clomid.

1. Call the clinic at the onset of your cycle.

2. You will typically have a sonogram on day 3, 4, or 5 of your cycle to make certain that you do not have any large cysts on your ovaries. If you have any existing cysts, they might be stimulated by Clomid, resulting in growth of the cyst and complications.

3. You will start urinary LH testing on approximately day 10 of your cycle, depending on your cycle's length. You should use your first morning urine for testing.

4. Once the urine test detects an LH surge, you should call the clinic before 2 p.m. that afternoon to schedule an insemination if you are using intrauterine insemination, or IUI (more on this later).

   Women who are not undergoing IUI should have intercourse the night the LH test turns positive and the following night. Doctor's orders!

quite expensive, to the tune of a few thousand dollars a month, so we encourage patients to consider using a reputable mail-order pharmacy that specializes in fertility medications. These drugs can cost 20 to 30 percent less by mail order than they do at a typical pharmacy.

Success rates for gonadotropins vary by age, but for a 35-year-old female with unexplained infertility, the success rates are about 15 to 17 percent per month, and approximately half of these pregnancies are for twins. The multiple birth rate is higher with use of gonadotropins than with Clomid.

Side Effects of Fertility Drugs

You may notice abdominal tenderness, bloating, fluid retention, and weight gain while you're taking fertility drugs. Women who take fertility drugs sometimes develop ovarian hyperstimulation syndrome (OHSS), a condition marked by weight gain and a full, bloated feeling. Some patients also experience shortness of breath, dizziness, pelvic pain, nausea, and vomiting.

Strangely, OHSS occurs when you respond too well to the drugs and produce too many eggs. Your ovaries rapidly swell to several times their size and leak fluid into your abdominal cavity. Normally this resolves itself and requires only careful monitoring by your physician. But in rare cases it can be life threatening, and you may have to be hospitalized for more intense monitoring.

Intrauterine Insemination

Intrauterine insemination (IUI) is a procedure in which a semen sample is washed, concentrated, and placed into the top of the uterine cavity with a thin catheter. This is basically a sperm limo service. More sperm are placed closer to the eggs so the little fellows have only half the distance to swim. Insemination is usually combined with an ovulation induction method.

Prior to insemination, the woman will undergo a hysterosalpingogram (HSG), an x-ray procedure (described in Chapter 2) to check for blockages or adhesions in her fallopian tubes.

IUI is most commonly used for infertility associated with endometriosis, unexplained infertility, infertility caused by ovulatory dysfunctions, very mild degrees of male-factor infertility, and cervical infertility.

It is not effective for patients with tubal blockage, severe tubal damage, very poor egg quantity and quality, ovarian failure (menopause), or severe male-factor infertility. IUI has only a small benefit for women who are over 40 years old, or for younger women with a significantly elevated day 3 FSH level. Those with other indications of significantly reduced ovarian reserve also will not derive much benefit from IUI. If the sperm count, motility, or morphology is more than slightly poor, insemination is quite unlikely to be successful.

A TYPICAL GONADOTROPIN TREATMENT CYCLE

1. Call your clinic before 5 p.m. on day 1 of your cycle. Day 1 is defined as the first day of menstrual flow that requires use of a pad or tampon.

2. You will have a vaginal sonogram and blood work, usually on day 2 or 3 of your cycle. This sonogram is performed to make certain that you do not have any large cysts on your ovaries that would prevent ovarian response to gonadotropins. Blood work is done to help determine the optimal dose of medication for you. Assuming these test results are within normal limits, you will start medication that evening. Remember to take your medication at approximately the same time each day.

3. You will return for blood work and sonograms after 2 to 4 days to determine how the ovaries are responding. You can expect between 3 to 5 sonograms with a gonadotropin cycle.

4. Once your follicles are mature, having grown to 15 to 20 millimeters in average diameter (we call them *oocytes* at this stage), gonadotropin is administered to induce ovulation. This injection is usually given between 9 p.m. and 11 p.m. If you are using IUI, you will have to abstain from sexual intercourse 2 to 5 days prior to insemination.

5. Insemination will be scheduled 36 hours after your gonadotropin injection. The insemination will take approximately 15 minutes. Good news: intercourse the night of the insemination and the following night is encouraged.

6. You will have a pregnancy test 12 to 14 days after insemination.

A TYPICAL INTRAUTERINE INSEMINATION PROCESS

1. You are typically given medication (either pills or injectable medications) to produce more than one egg. (See discussion of ovulation induction on page 40.) The insemination is then timed to coincide with ovulation.

2. You will undergo tests—either urinary LH testing (for Clomid) or ultrasound and blood tests (for fertility injections)—to determine when ovulation will occur.

3. Your partner will produce a semen specimen either at home or at the clinic after (ideally) 2 to 5 days of abstinence from ejaculation. The semen is "washed" in the laboratory. In this process, the sperm are separated from the other components of the semen and concentrated in a small volume. Various techniques can be used to perform the washing and separation, depending on the specifics of the individual case and preferences of the laboratory. The sperm processing takes about 40 to 60 minutes.

4. The separated and washed sperm specimen, consisting of a purified fraction of highly motile sperm, is placed high in the uterine cavity using a very thin, soft catheter.

5. We will ask you to remain lying down for 10 minutes following the procedure. As the sperm specimen is above the level of the vagina, it will not leak out when you stand up.

6. This procedure typically feels similar to a Pap smear. There should be little or no discomfort. Some mild uterine cramping occasionally occurs.

In Vitro Fertilization

In vitro fertilization (IVF) is a process in which a woman's ovaries are stimulated by a series of hormone shots, causing the ovaries to produce multiple eggs. These eggs are then "harvested" or retrieved from the ovaries. The retrieval is a minor surgical procedure in which the physician inserts a needle into the ovaries through the vagina using an ultrasound image for guidance.

After the eggs are retrieved, the embryologist prepares them for fertilization. The sperm is then used to fertilize the eggs either via natural fertilization or by a procedure called intracytoplasmic sperm injection (ICSI), in which a single sperm is injected into each egg.

After fertilization, the embryos are cultured in the IVF lab. A select number of embryos are then chosen and transferred to the uterus similar to a Pap smear.

Ovarian Stimulation

During this very important phase of the IVF cycle, gonadotropins are administered (as with ovulation induction) to stimulate the ovaries to produce multiple eggs. The stimulation phase of the cycle lasts on average 10 days, but can often vary from 8 to 12 days.

The ovarian response to these medications is monitored by measuring levels of estradiol in the blood and by observing the ovaries via vaginal ultrasound. Once the ovaries appear ready to undergo egg retrieval, an injection of human chorionic gonadotropin is given to bring the eggs to final maturity. The egg retrieval is typically scheduled 35 hours after the gonadotropin injection.

Other medications administered might include steroids and a medication to prevent ovulation. Steroids are given to block a rise in male hormone levels which in turn helps egg development. A drug to prevent ovulation is given so that the eggs are not released before the retrieval can occur.

Egg Retrieval

Follicles are sacs of fluid that contain eggs, or *oocytes*. When the follicles reach 15 to 20 millimeters in diameter, the egg is ripe and ready to be retrieved. A needle is inserted into the follicle to suck out the fluid. The egg floats out with the fluid down the needle into a test tube. This procedure is performed with the physician using an ultrasound image to guide the needle. The patient is under IV sedation. After the retrieval, the embryologist will identify the eggs in the follicular fluid under a microscope. The procedure typically takes about 10 to 20 minutes and is performed in an outpatient surgical setting.

Insemination

After egg retrieval, the eggs are fertilized. They are cultured for 3 to 5 days, and then they are ready for transfer into the uterus. At this stage, they are between 8 and 60 cells in size.

A TYPICAL IVF CYCLE

1. You will have your initial consultation with the physician.

2. You will complete your IVF workup. An IVF workup typically includes a baseline vaginal ultrasound, an office hysteroscopy (to evaluate the uterine cavity), a mock trial embryo transfer, a semen analysis on your partner (if applicable), and lab work. The lab typically includes genetic testing, blood type/antibody testing, communicable disease testing, as well as other patient specific testing recommended by your physician.

3. Once the results of your lab work and testing are completed and reviewed by the physician, the physician will make recommendations for your personal protocol that will be used for your IVF cycle. It is after all of your workup and testing has been completed that your IVF calendar will be initiated.

4. You will attend an IVF teaching visit with one of the nurses. Medication will be prescribed, and instructions on how to administer your medications as well as detailed instructions on your calendar will be reviewed during this visit. You will be given copies of the consents and have the opportunity to discuss the contents of the consents and clarify any questions you might have.

5. Many of the calendar protocols will be initiated with the start of the birth control pill. Birth control pills are started to avoid the formation of ovarian cysts and to make the timing of the start of the fertility drugs easier. The baseline sonogram shows whether the ovaries and uterus look normal before beginning the medications. Prior to stimulation of the ovary a suppression ultrasound check will be completed. This is important to ensure that there are no cysts currently active on your ovaries.

6. Ovarian stimulation medications will be initiated.

7. Regular morning ultrasounds and lab work will be performed to adjust your medication dosages and determine when the follicles are mature.

8. Egg retrieval is performed.

9. Embryo transfer procedure is performed.

10. A pregnancy blood test is performed 14 days after your egg retrieval date.

Embryo Transfer

The embryo transfer is done 3 to 5 days after egg retrieval. The physician performing the transfer will discuss with you and your partner the status of your embryos and the number to be transferred. The number of embryos transferred will vary according to their quality. You will be offered the opportunity to freeze any remaining embryos that are of high quality. The transfer is a process similar to that of a Pap smear. The transfer is easy and virtually pain free in most cases. Following transfer, most centers require bed rest for the day of transfer and the following day. Two weeks after the egg retrieval, you will take a pregnancy test.

In this and the first two chapters, I've provided you with the basic and general information you'll need to ask the right questions, serve as your own best advocate, and take the proper steps to help identify your particular infertility challenges.

In the next six chapters, I offer much more specific information pertaining to the most common diagnoses for infertility patients. You are free to read just those that apply to you or your partner, or any that interest you. It is not uncommon for infertility patients to have more than one challenge, so you may find the other chapters useful. The goal of each chapter is to give you all the information you need to ask the right questions and to feel in control as you fight for your fertility. You should also take hope from this information because we've come a long way in treating these common causes of infertility. Even in the most complex cases, we are often able to find ways to help our patients achieve their goals of starting a family.

Part II

The Most
Common Fertility
Challenges

CHAPTER FOUR

Polycystic Ovary Syndrome

JANE, 32, HAD been taking a fertility drug prescribed by her gynecologist for a year, but without success, even after he upped it, first to two and then to three pills a day.

Our staff did the full workup of tests and examinations for Jane and her husband, Victor, and the true source of her infertility quickly became apparent. Jane had experienced irregular menstruation since her teenage years. She often went months without having a period. This problem was masked for many years because she was put on birth control pills as a teen to regulate her cycles. She stayed on them until her late twenties.

As soon as she stopped taking the pill, Jane again found that her cycles were irregular. She also began to gain weight regardless of how much she ate. "I store everything, like a squirrel," she said. Jane was disturbed also that she suddenly was experiencing acne and extra hair growth.

Irregular cycles, infertility, weight gain, acne, and hair growth may seem like unrelated problems—and unfortunately, many family doctors and OB-GYNs come to that conclusion. The fact is that when they occur together, they are classic signs of *polycystic ovary syndrome* (PCOS).

PCOS is one of the most common causes of ovulation disorders. If you have symptoms similar to Jane's—lack of ovulation, excess hair growth, acne, or unexplained weight gain or obesity—you should read this chapter. If the underlying cause of your symptoms is PCOS, an accurate diagnosis and effective treatment could truly change your life. Besides helping you conquer your infertility, there are lifelong risks associated with PCOS that can be mitigated with simple treatment.

In addition to her symptoms, there were other telltale signs of PCOS in Jane's case. While performing an ultrasound examination for Jane, we found that her uterus and tubes were normal—a good sign—but we detected multiple small follicles in the ovary. These typically resemble a ring of pearls on a necklace and are indicative of PCOS. We also measured Jane's insulin and glucose levels and they were abnormal. It is common for patients with PCOS to have insulin resistance.

Fortunately, there are proven treatments for this very common cause of infertility. Since Jane's husband had normal sperm tests, and her uterus and tubes were healthy, we knew that there was a good chance for this couple to have children.

For Jane, we prescribed metformin, a drug used to treat diabetics because it improves the use of insulin in the body. We then put Jane on a lower dose of Clomid—the same drug her gynecologist had prescribed—and, thanks also to the metformin, she ovulated. Because the high doses of Clomid she had taken previously had dried up her cervical mucus (a common side effect), we performed intrauterine insemination (IUI). On the very first cycle of metformin, Clomid, and insemination, Jane conceived. She delivered a healthy girl nine months later.

Then, several months after her baby was born, Jane, who hoped to have another child in a few years, returned to our clinic to discuss her ongoing concern about her irregular cycles and her propensity for weight gain, acne, and hair growth.

We put her back on metformin, which improved her body's production and use of insulin. This in turn lowered her male hormone production and helped her control her weight, acne, and hair growth. She was also placed on birth control pills to further suppress her male hormones and give her regular menstrual cycles.

This treatment has remarkably improved Jane's quality of life. It has kept her body in a more normal state of hormone balance until she is ready for a second baby.

There are several lessons to be drawn from Jane's PCOS case. Some patients are placed on Clomid for very long periods by their general OB-GYNs or physicians when it is evident that patients are not likely to become pregnant if they haven't already done so after three to four cycles of Clomid. These patients, therefore, should be referred to a specialist for further evaluation after a maximum of four Clomid cycles.

Jane's case also illustrates that although Clomid can successfully produce ovulation, it often dries up the cervical mucus, which means that without intrauterine insemination, pregnancy is less likely to occur. And finally, Jane is a star patient because she followed through and continued to get treatment after she had children, which has ensured she will be healthy enough to care for and enjoy them as they grow.

Polycystic Ovary Syndrome and You

Women with PCOS often have irregular cycles beginning in puberty. This syndrome has been found in girls as young as 8 years of age. If an adolescent's menstrual cycles have not become regular 2 to 3 years after her first period, there is a strong possibility that she might have PCOS.

Unfortunately, it is estimated that at least 70 percent of PCOS cases are not diagnosed. Often young women complain of irregular menstrual cycles only to be told it is "normal" or the result of "stress." They are then given birth control pills to cover up the symptoms and make their cycles regular. But that only masks the problem until they get off birth control and try to get pregnant. As a result, many cases are diagnosed only when a patient has difficulty conceiving. Yet the earlier that PCOS is diagnosed, the higher the likelihood that the signs and symptoms can be controlled, long-term health risks can be avoided, and for some, ovulatory function can be maintained.

PCOS can come with a variety of symptoms, none of them pleasant. In addition to menstrual dysfunction, patients often complain of symptoms related to excess male hormones. Typical clinical symptoms include acne; hair growth on the face, stomach and back; and occasionally, male pattern balding.

These symptoms occur when the ovarian tissue converts male hormones (androgens), which occur at higher levels in PCOS patients, to testosterone. The pituitary in PCOS patients secretes more luteinizing hormone (LH), which stimulates the enlarged ovaries to produce more testosterone. Elevated male hormones can often be measured in the blood of patients with PCOS. These excess hormones cause undesirable changes in the body, including weight gain, acne, and increased facial and body hair.

PCOS is associated with insulin resistance. In fact, many patients will have a family history of diabetes. PCOS patients often have *acanthosis nigricans*, a dark thickening of the skin at the nape of the neck, armpits, and groin area with small finger like protrusions of extra skin. These "skin tags" are only a cosmetic issue. This symptom is a hallmark of insulin resistance. Approximately 30 percent of overweight PCOS patients will eventually develop diabetes. PCOS worsens with weight gain.

Thin patients with PCOS can also display abnormal insulin release in response to a sugar load, but may not complain of acne and facial hair because they have lower androgen levels. A lean PCOS patient may also gain significant amounts of weight and eventually present as a classic PCOS case; therefore, exercise and proper nutrition are important. I can't emphasize that enough, because when a woman has PCOS, her androgen and insulin secre-

SIGNS AND SYMPTOMS OF POLYCYSTIC OVARY SYNDROME (PSOS)

○ Irregular cycles

○ Lack of ovulation

○ Infertility

○ Multifollicular ovaries
(12 or more follicles
in at least one ovary)

○ Insulin resistance

○ Obesity

○ Excess male hormone
levels leading to abnormal
hair growth, male pattern
balding, acne

tion will worsen as her weight increases, making it less likely that she will conceive.

Some of the symptoms associated with PCOS may also indicate ovulatory dysfunction. Careful diagnosis is critical because the treatments for the two conditions vary. For example, women with eating disorders, women who exercise excessively, and women with low body mass index (BMI) may actually have ovulatory dysfunction. They also may have what appear to be polycystic ovaries on ultrasound, yet they will not complain of issues such as acne and hair growth, and they will have normal testosterone levels.

Diagnosing Polycystic Ovary Syndrome

Ultrasound is a great way to check for PCOS. The ovaries of PCOS patients have more follicles than normal. They often form a ring around the outside of the ovary, creating the appearance of a chain of pearls. Twelve or more follicles in each ovary is a sign of polycystic ovaries.

To reach a correct diagnosis of PCOS, other conditions such as thyroid problems, elevated prolactin secretion, and other rare hormonal conditions must be ruled out. In addition, two out of the following three criteria must be present for the diagnosis of PCOS:

○ Irregular cycles

○ Unusual hair growth, acne, hair loss, or balding (with or without laboratory evidence of elevated testosterone levels)

○ The presence of 12 or more follicles on each ovary

Testing for Polycystic Ovary Syndrome

During the initial visit, a patient who suspects PCOS should have a thorough physical exam, paying special attention to any unusual hair growth and presence of dark, thick, velvety skin in the armpits, groin, and neck. An ultrasound should be performed to assess the appearance of the ovaries and to look for excess follicles.

Blood tests should also be done to detect metabolic problems associated with PCOS, such as increased glucose levels and lipids. These tests can determine which patients need special diets or medications to minimize the risk of diabetes and cardiovascular disease. The patient should fast the night before the tests, ingesting nothing after midnight except water. For couples trying to conceive, it is also essential to complete the necessary infertility testing, such as a semen analysis for the male partner and an x-ray examination of the uterus and fallopian tubes, before beginning treatment for PCOS. Patients who are overweight or have impaired glucose tolerance should see a nutritionist and exercise at least five times per week for at least 30 to 40 minutes.

For the diabetic patient, glucose levels must be well controlled. Hemoglobin A1C, which is a measure of elevated glucose levels in the blood, should be approximately six or under before conception. A higher risk for miscarriage and severe birth defects may result if these levels are not well controlled. A decrease in as little as 5 to 10 percent of body weight can re-initiate ovulatory cycles.

Research by nutritional experts and others has shown that low carbohydrate diets and low calorie diets work equally well for decreasing weight. There is concern, however, that diets that restrict carbohydrates are difficult to maintain. Most patients regain the weight lost and sometimes gain additional weight. (In sheep, carbohydrate restriction compromises fertility potential.)

Our patient Donna had a history of irregular menstrual cycles. She thought it nothing unusual that her cycles came every 35 to 50 days. In fact, she considered it a blessing that she didn't have to deal with monthly bloating, breast tenderness, or premenstrual symptoms.

Then, at the age of 20, Donna began to notice the occasional facial hair that required plucking. She also had difficulty maintaining her weight. By her early thirties, Donna's weight had ballooned to 208 pounds and she was shaving facial hair every 2 weeks.

Her symptoms were classic, so it was no surprise that at her first appointment with a reproductive endocrinologist, Donna was diagnosed with PCOS. After numerous metabolic tests, Donna learned that not only had her weight impeded her ability to conceive, it also put her at risk for developing diabetes.

She wisely enrolled in a nutritional program, and once she began exercising each week, Donna lost 20 pounds. Because of her difficulty metabolizing glucose, Donna began taking metformin, the insulin sensitizing drug used to treat diabetics. Slowly, her cycles normalized to every 35 days. Blood testing indicated that she was ovulating. Her physician still recommended that she use Clomid, and within 3 months Donna had a positive pregnancy test. During her pregnancy, Donna was screened multiple times for diabetes, but always passed her tests.

Donna delivered a healthy baby boy while experiencing only a slight increase in her blood pressure. Unfortunately, Donna was unable to lose the "baby weight," and by the time she returned for treatment 2 years later, her tests were abnormal and her cholesterol was elevated. But after a year of conscientious lifestyle changes, Donna dropped her weight to under 170 pounds. She conceived her second child naturally.

It's troubling for fertility doctors when a patient doesn't continue to take care of herself after delivering a baby. Far too many PCOS patients fall off the wagon. They do not continue to address the associated long-term health concerns associated with this syndrome, such as diabetes, heart disease, and endometrial cancer. Because of the weight and cosmetic issues, PCOS patients can also suffer from poor self-confidence and depression. Assistance from other health care professionals such as therapists and nutritionists allow the medical team to better serve PCOS patients.

Weight Reduction Can Help Fertility

Losing just 5 to 10 percent of your body weight can help jump-start your ovulatory cycles. But remember to reduce your weight the smart way. Control portion size and eat low-fat foods with sufficient protein and complex carbohydrates. The key strategy for PCOS patients is a *change in lifestyle.* You should choose a nutritional or exercise program that you can stick to for the rest of your life. There are numerous studies in Europe and the United States which show that a more fit and active lifestyle combined with healthy nutritional choices can decrease the incidence of diabetes in insulin-resistant patients by as much as 61 percent. Unfortunately, this lifestyle is difficult for many patients to sustain, and nearly 95 percent of those who lose weight will gain it back if not given continued medical and emotional support.

Once you've gone through your initial examination and diagnosis, you and your physician must decide whether it would be beneficial to delay conception for 6 to 12 months while you modify your lifestyle. It might be that other factors, such as the patient's age, argue for initiating therapy quickly. For patients who are extremely overweight, surgical techniques such as laparoscopic banding or gastric bypass may be an option. Women who undergo these extreme measures can reverse the insulin resistance, halt the high blood pressure associated with being overweight, and increase their probability of ovulation. In addition, there have been several studies that have shown a decrease in birth defects and lower rates of gestational diabetes in women who have successfully lost weight.

Fertility Treatments for Polycystic Ovary Syndrome

Clomid

For patients who proceed quickly with treatment rather than waiting to lose weight, studies have shown that ovulation induction with Clomid should be the first line of treatment. Clomid is a stealth medication that tricks your body into releasing the follicle-stimulating hormone (FSH) needed to help you conceive. It works in the part of the brain known as the hypothalamus, which is the regulatory center for the pituitary. The hypothalamus induces the pituitary gland to release more FSH, which in turn drives ovarian follicular development.

The starting dose of Clomid is often 50 milligrams. It is not uncommon to start as high as 100 milligrams if a patient is overweight. If a patient has not had a period, progesterone may be given to induce it before beginning a course of Clomid.

As the dose of Clomid increases, there can be a negative effect on the endometrium. Higher doses of Clomid can shrink the endometrium. The thinner the endometrial wall, the lower the probability of implantation, and, hence, of pregnancy. In addition, high doses of Clomid hinder the production of cervical mucus, which can diminish sperm motility.

Patients are instructed to begin using urine ovulation kits on the third day after the last pill. A positive ovulation surge will be detected 5 to 12 days after the last tablet. An ultrasound is often performed during this time to assess follicular response and the thickness of the endometrium.

Clomid is started on day 2 to 5 of the menstrual cycle and is taken for 5 days. Patients are instructed to begin using urine-testing ovulation kits on the third day after the last pill. A positive ovulation surge will be detected 5 to 12 days after the patient has taken the last pill. An ultrasound is often performed during this time to assess the follicular response and the thickness of the endometrium.

If an ovulation surge has not occurred spontaneously, an injection of human chorionic gonadotropin (hCG) can be administered to induce ovulation once a follicle has grown to 20 millimeters. Ovulation should occur within 36 to 42 hours, at which time the couple should have intercourse.

Patients will continue this regimen for a total of three to six cycles. If they are unsuccessful, intrauterine insemination is added. Although couples may be frustrated at this point, the good news is that pregnancy rates reach 70 to 75 percent over six to nine cycles of treatment.

Most PCOS patients will respond to 50 or 100 milligrams of Clomid. If ovulation does not occur, the dose of Clomid can be increased to 200 milligrams; however, only 7 percent of patients will ovulate at this dose. If such a high dose is required, it is best to consider other therapies, such as the addition of metformin or gonadotropins. Still, as I've noted, increasing doses of Clomid can impair implantation by affecting the endometrium and can hamper normal cervical mucus function.

Metformin

For the patient with a known history of impaired glucose tolerance or diabetes, most experts agree that an insulin sensitizer such as metformin should be started prior to initiating treatment. Metformin was approved for the treatment of type II diabetes by the FDA in 1994; however, it was widely used for more than 30 years in other parts of the world. Metformin works primarily by suppressing glucose production in the liver but also improves insulin sensitivity in the periphery. Gastrointestinal symptoms, such as diarrhea, nausea, abdominal bloating, and flatulence, are the most common side effects.

There is a small risk of accumulating lactic acid in patients taking metformin, but this occurs more commonly in patients with poorly controlled diabetes and impaired renal function. Still, for safety reasons, metformin should be discontinued the day prior to any intravenous radiologic procedures such as a hysterosalpingogram (HSG).

There have been no reported fetal abnormalities associated with the use of metformin in women with diabetes or PCOS who have taken this drug while pregnant. Studies have shown that optimal dosing is 1,500 milligrams to 2,550 milligrams per day.

At one time, it was common to start PCOS patients of all weights on metformin before attempting Clomid. However, there have been trials showing no difference in pregnancy rates in patients taking Clomid versus Clomid in combination with metformin. Interestingly, studies have shown a higher ovulation response in the combination group. Other questions, such as whether there is a decrease in gestational diabetes or miscarriage, have not been addressed.

Patients who wish to lose weight before treatment have been shown to benefit from metformin, which is typically started up to 6 months before attempting conception. Among such women, more than 60 percent had improved cycles and ovulation, and more than 80 percent achieved regular cycles. Patients who resume regular cycles and can detect ovulation can avoid Clomid altogether and thus decrease their risk of multiple births.

Another option currently receiving a great deal of attention is the reduction in miscarriage rates with the use of metformin. Elevated levels of insulin interfere with the normal balance between factors promoting blood clotting and those promoting breakdown of the clots. This imbalance may result in abnormal development in the endometrium and placenta, eventually compromising blood flow to the fetus, leading to miscarriage.

Retrospective studies have reported that metformin decreased the risk of miscarriage in PCOS patients from approximately 40 percent to 10 percent. However, we should note that another study found a 35 percent miscarriage rate in 20 pregnancies treated with metformin through 12 weeks of gestation.

Gonadotropins

One option for PCOS patients who fail to ovulate despite metformin and Clomid therapy is to be treated with low-dose gonadotropins. Gonadotropins contain FSH and other combinations of FSH and luteinizing hormone (LH).

With low-dose gonadotropins (that is, at dosages of 37.5 milligrams to 75 milligrams per day), about 95 percent of patients will ovulate, with a 55 percent cumulative pregnancy rate after six cycles. In other words, once they achieve ovulation, approximately half of the patients will eventually conceive. Overall, in women with PCOS but without other infertility factors, about 88 percent of those ovulating will eventually conceive, with a conception rate of 22 percent per month per single cycle or ovulation or single attempt with drugs and IUI. The 88 percent rate is after the patient tries many cycles and is either pregnant or gives up; it could be 3, 4, 6, or more attempts. Probability is not additive so it never reaches 100 percent; that is, 12 percent never conceive no matter how long they try.

Some PCOS patients, despite the use of low-dose gonadotropins, can develop multiple follicles, placing them at risk for bearing triplets or more. There is also a significant probability of ovarian hyperstimulation syndrome, which is characterized by the presence of multiple cysts within the ovaries. This condition can lead to ovarian enlargement and other complications.

When there is a high risk of hyperstimulation, the cycle should be cancelled, or it should be converted to in vitro fertilization, in which case the number of embryos transferred can be limited. There is no justification for a patient having high-order multiple births (triplets or more). There have been studies indicating that initiating metformin at least 6 to 8 weeks before the use of gonadotropins or IVF may allow for a more controlled stimulation of the ovaries, decreasing the risk of multiples. Other studies of the same treatment have reported even better egg quality and embryo development and excellent pregnancy rates. However, a number of similar studies have shown no benefit; therefore, more research is needed to address these issues.

Ovarian Diathermy

There also has been renewed interest in the surgical alternative to inducing ovulation in women with PCOS using a procedure called *ovarian diathermy*. During this procedure, a laser fiber or electrosurgical needle is used to produce multiple burns in the ovarian capsule. This treatment destroys the ovarian tissue that produces androgens and thus reduces testosterone levels. Studies have shown that patients who do not respond to Clomid have ovulatory response rates as high as 80 percent with ovarian diathermy.

Unfortunately, the ovulatory response is short-lived and most women return to anovulatory cycles (that is, cycles without ovulation) after 8 months. Moreover, ovarian diathermy is associated with severe adhesion formation, or scar tissue, around the ovaries and tubes, which can actually worsen infertility by preventing the egg from traveling to the fallopian tube. Thus, the risks associated with this procedure significantly limit its use.

The In Vitro Option

For women with PCOS who can't be treated by traditional therapy and require in vitro fertilization (IVF), success rates are quite high, approaching 60 to 70 percent delivery rates at our clinic. (IVF is discussed in depth in Chapter 12.) The obstacles that PCOS patients must typically surmount when they undergo IVF include higher numbers of immature eggs, abnormal embryo development, and the risk of ovarian hyperstimulation, which is characterized by the presence of multiple cysts within the ovaries.

Your doctor should take particular care to avoid ovarian hyperstimulation. When ovarian hyperstimulation syndrome occurs, fluid can accumulate in the abdomen causing distension, nausea, and shortness of breath. Patients will then

TREATMENT OPTIONS FOR PSOS

○ Weight loss
○ Metformin
  (Glucophage®)
○ In vitro fertilization

○ Clomiphene citrate
  (Clomid®)
○ Gonadotropins (FSH)

experience vomiting and diarrhea, which further aggravate the syndrome. Some patients (less than 1 percent) will require hospitalization. All the above symptoms are interlinked and result from doctors being too aggressive. Ovarian hyperstimulation can occur when a doctor uses high doses of gonadotropins for stimulation, opts not to administer metformin, and retrieves the eggs before the follicular size is appropriate.

One proven method to control the stimulation response and address these issues is to administer oral contraceptives for several weeks before initiating an IVF cycle. The effectiveness of this strategy has been documented time and time again. There are other ways to reduce this risk as well. Your doctors may decrease the initial dose of the fertility injections, increasing the dosage only slowly and only if needed. Another strategy is to lower the dose of human chorionic gonadotropins used in IVF cycles to promote maturity of the eggs before retrieval. Your doctor might also use Lupron (leuprolide acetate) to induce egg maturity.

More than 3 million women in the United States have PCOS. Of those, it is estimated that 1 million are diabetic, even at a young age. Women who are experiencing any of the symptoms associated with PCOS need to understand that early intervention can significantly change the course of this syndrome. Early treatments coupled with nutritional education and exercise can improve fertility and decrease long-term health risks.

PCOS patients generally have an excellent chance of becoming pregnant with therapy. It's not always easy because the treatments may be complex and time consuming, but as many of our patients who never thought they'd be able to have children say, when things go right, it's worth all of the effort.

Chapter Five

Endometriosis and Its Impact on Fertility

Diane, 33, tried to get pregnant for 3 years with her husband, Jeff. Both were in excellent health. Diane took prenatal vitamins religiously after going off birth control pills. She noticed that her periods became more and more painful a few months after she stopped taking her contraceptive. She'd also experienced pain during intercourse, which had never happened when she was on the pill.

Worried, Diane consulted with her gynecologist, who performed a physical and an ultrasound examination. Diane experienced some pelvic tenderness with both exams. The gynecologist called in Jeff, too, and the couple underwent a range of tests that included a semen analysis for him and an HSG (hystero-salpingogram) x-ray exam of Diane's uterus, fallopian tubes, and the surrounding areas. The tests also included basic blood work. All the test results were normal.

Diane's doctor suspected endometriosis was the cause of her painful periods and the pain she felt during sex. Endometriosis is also a common cause of infertility. It occurs when microscopic particles of uterine glandular tissue (endometrium) migrate backwards through the fallopian tubes then implant and grow in places they do not belong, causing inflammation, which results in pain and infertility.

Increasingly painful periods and pain during sex are the most common symptoms, but many women may experience pain at other times as well.

For example, some women experience pain during bowel movements and urination. The prevalence of this disease in the general population varies from 2 to nearly 8 percent, but it is much more common in women with chronic pelvic pain.

What Is Endometriosis and What Does It Do?

Endometriosis is usually not life-threatening, but it is a serious and complex disease that medical researchers are still trying to understand fully. This disease primarily affects the reproductive organs and pelvic region of a woman's body. It gets its name from its similarity to the lining of the womb, or endometrium. This disease will start without noticeable symptoms, then gradually the patient will notice painful periods and increasing amounts of pain during sex. Rapid progression will often occur when a woman discontinues birth control pills in an effort to conceive.

Microscopic uterine glandular tissue, similar to the endometrium, or lining of the womb, finds its way into the pelvic cavity and subsequently implants on healthy tissue there. These particles of tissue behave in the same manner as the endometrium. The natural activity of the endometrium is to respond to hormones produced by the ovaries so that each month the glands and other tissue within the endometrium build up to prepare for pregnancy. When pregnancy does not occur, the endometrial lining is shed, and women have a period.

A similar reaction takes place in the stray cells that have found their way into the pelvic cavity. Each month they react to hormones, and break down, and bleed, but the blood and tissue shed from these endometrial growths have no way of leaving the body. This results in internal bleeding, and the breakdown of the blood and tissue from these sites leads to inflammation.

This process continues for months or even years before symptoms of serious pain begin to develop. Many women start to suspect something is wrong because the amount of pain they feel with their periods starts to get worse and worse as the months go by.

For other women, the disease may not manifest any noticeable symptoms, but they may have difficulty conceiving. It is then that they seek medical advice, which could lead to a diagnosis by laparoscopy.

If untreated, this disease may progress and start to do more damage in the pelvic cavity. Eventually it can lead to adhesions (scar tissue), chronic pelvic pain, bowel and urinary problems, and infertility, as well as a gradual decline in general health. Implanted endometrial tissue can be present on the intestines, diaphragm, liver surface, surgical scars, and even on the surface of the lung (although this is extremely rare). It is also important to note that sometimes endometriosis does not progress at all and may not cause any painful symptoms or infertility.

Endometriosis in Context

Endometriosis is serious. It affects millions of women around the world. It can be a devastating disorder, affecting women's health, quality of life, fertility, emotional well-being, sex life, and relationships.

Endometriosis is not usually fatal, though there may be rare occasions when the symptoms can pose a serious threat to a patient's life. It is not a disease that you catch from another person. Basically, it appears to be a defect in the body's natural healing processes. It can strike women at any time of their reproductive life, but we are seeing more and more cases among teenagers.

Recent studies indicate that women with the disease are at greater risk of having other health problems, but this correlation may indicate that women with endometriosis are actually suffering from a breakdown in the immune system. This hypothesis seems to ring true, as many women who have endometriosis seem to suffer from a myriad of other health problems.

The complexity of this disease is reflected in a recent study that found almost two-thirds of women with a diagnosis of endometriosis had previously been told by a physician that nothing was wrong. Other studies have offered the alarming fact that the median delay in diagnosis can be more than 8 years.

Although pelvic pain and infertility are classic symptoms of endometriosis, it is important to understand that there are other abnormalities, including prior pelvic infection, scar tissue, and urologic or gastroenterological conditions, that can cause similar symptoms.

Studies have shown that a woman with endometriosis is 10 to 17 percent more likely to have difficulty conceiving. Symptoms from endometriosis typically peak in women in their mid-twenties but can occur in adolescents as well. It is very common for pain to become progressively worse after women who wish to conceive stop their oral contraceptives.

Complexities of Endometriosis

Research has found that alterations in the immune system and the chemistry of the abdominal cavity may play major roles in the establishment and proliferation of this complex disease. The fluid within the abdominal cavity in women with endometriosis may actually have a toxic effect on embryos. Endometriosis may also interfere with the proteins involved with embryo implantation, which would also adversely affect fertility.

The end stage of this disorder's inflammatory process results in scar tissue (adhesions), which can close the fallopian tubes, prevent the tube from picking up the egg at the time of ovulation, or make the ovary inaccessible to the fallopian tubes.

Diagnosing Endometriosis

Unfortunately, there is not a single simple way to diagnose endometriosis, which can be frustrating for patients. Symptoms and physical examination are a good start, but are not precise, so further confirmation is required. Pelvic ultrasound exams may reveal ovarian masses suggestive of an *endometrioma*, also known as a chocolate cyst, but this finding should not be relied upon for a definitive diagnosis. These are cysts lined by endometriosis. Monthly bleeding into the cyst from the endometrial tissue fills it with red or brown blood. Depending on their size, these cysts can cause pain, and they can interfere with follicular development and ovulation.

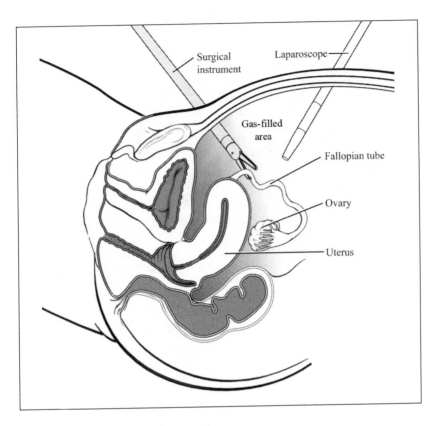

Surgical instrument

Laparoscope

Gas-filled area

Fallopian tube

Ovary

Uterus

Figure 1: Laparascopic procedure

The ultrasound will not reveal the implants typically associated with endometriosis. Researchers have tried to create reliable diagnostic tests of the blood or uterine lining, but so far none have been approved. The best method for diagnosing and surgically treating endometriosis is *laparoscopy*. It is typically performed under general anesthesia on an outpatient basis. A small incision is made below the belly button, and a small tube with very small camera is threaded inside. One to three additional incisions are made in the pubic hair line, through which instruments are introduced (see Figure 1). In this way, the pelvis can be inspected for endometriosis, pelvic adhesions, and structural abnormalities in the fallopian tubes or ovaries.

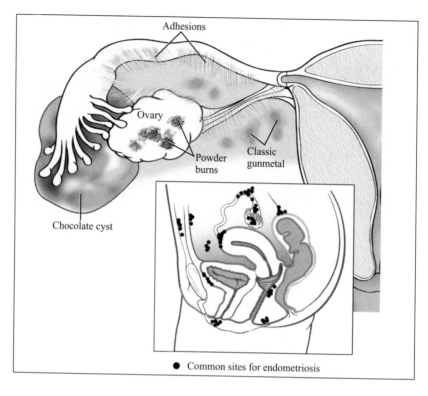

Adhesions

Ovary

Powder
burns

Classic
gunmetal

Chocolate cyst

● Common sites for endometriosis

Figure 2: Characteristics of endometriosis

Endometriosis has several distinctive visual characteristics, including bright red or "flame" lesions, black or "powder burn" lesions, scar tissue or "white" lesions, nodules, vesicular or "clear" lesions, and, as mentioned earlier, endometriomas or chocolate cysts (see Figure 2).

In our patient Diane's case, the gynecologist recommended that a laparoscopy be performed. During the laparoscopy on Diane, her doctor found stage II (mild) endometriosis on the surface of her bladder and pelvis, with normal looking fallopian tubes and ovaries. Using a laser, he treated all the disease that he could see.

Because of the particular challenges posed by endometriosis, you should

	ENDOMETRIOSIS	<1CM	1–3CM	>3CM
PERITONEUM	Superficial	1	2	4
	Deep	2	4	6
OVARY	R Superficial	1	2	4
	Deep	4	16	20
	L Superficial	1	2	4
	Deep	4	16	20

POSTERIOR CULDESAC OBLITERATION	PARTIAL	COMPLETE
	4	40

	ADHESIONS	<⅓ ENCLOSURE	⅓–⅔ ENCLOSURE	>⅔ ENCLOSURE
OVARY	R Filmy	1	2	4
	Dense	4	8	16
	L Filmy	1	2	4
	Dense	4	8	16
TUBE	R Filmy	1	2	4
	Dense	4	8	16
	L Filmy	1	2	4
	Dense	4	8	16

Stage I (Minimal)—1–5
Stage II (Mild)—6–15
Stage III (Moderate)—16–40
Stage IV (Severe)—>40
Total_____

Figure 3: The American Society for Reproductive Medicine's revised classification of endometriosis

choose a surgeon with a special expertise treating it. The American Society for Reproductive Medicine (ASRM) has developed a staging or rating system for the severity of this disorder based on laparoscopic findings. This rating system is used to measure the potential for pregnancy (see Figure 3). Keep in mind, however, that this rating system is highly subjective and might not accurately predict whether a woman will become pregnant.

What You Need to Know about Surgical Treatments

Make certain that you have chosen a surgeon who is prepared to treat most forms of endometriosis at the time of the initial laparoscopy. This will minimize the need for a second operation. Keep in mind, however, that there is no one correct way to treat this disease surgically. Skilled surgeons will use a variety of approaches, including *excision* (cutting out) or *ablation* (destroying) of lesions. The latter approach can be accomplished with lasers, high-intensity ultrasound, and electrical energy sources. The goal is to not only remove as much of the endometriosis tissue as possible but to restore your anatomy to as normal a state as possible and to minimize the development of new scar tissue.

Some studies have suggested that neither treatment, excision or ablation, is better with respect to fertility. However, the largest study of this condition suggests that ablation is the better method. Doctors in Canada evaluated 341 patients with less extensive endometriosis. Pregnancy rates were significantly higher in the group treated with ablation (37.5 percent versus 22.5 percent), and their pregnancies were achieved more rapidly as well. However, the monthly overall pregnancy rates were still low: 4.7 percent versus 2.4 percent.

As you might expect, surgical treatment of endometriosis is more challenging and can be much more extensive in the advanced stages of the disease. When performed by a skilled laparoscopic surgeon, these procedures can be very effective at eradicating painful symptoms. But they will improve fertility only if the normal functions between the tubes and ovaries can be restored and relevant scar tissue removed.

When an endometrioma (chocolate cyst) is identified, the surgeon may either drain or remove the cyst. Studies show that recurrence rates were significantly lower and spontaneous pregnancy rates were significantly higher with excision of the cyst capsule as opposed to drainage, although the latter is a much easier procedure to perform. It is critical that the surgeon take great care to preserve surrounding normal ovarian tissue and blood supply when removing the cyst capsule so as not to compromise ovarian reserve.

Certain drugs suppress the hormones that appear to stimulate the spread of endometriosis and help alleviate the pain associated with this disease. These include oral contraceptives, progestins (synthetic derivatives of progesterone), danazol (a synthetic derivative of testosterone), and gonadotropin-releasing hormone (GnRH) agonists (drugs that block the pituitary from releasing LH and causing premature ovulation). While these are helpful in decreasing pain, they've not been shown to help women become pregnant on their own.

Fertility Drugs and Intrauterine Insemination

Fertility drugs such as clomiphene citrate (Clomid) or gonadotropins, coupled with intrauterine insemination (IUI), can help women whose fertility is affected by endometriosis, as long as there is at least one fallopian tube that is open and normal, and as long as there is no significant distortion of her pelvic anatomy.

Our patient Diane and her husband elected to undergo an initial course of treatment with Clomid and intrauterine insemination (IUI) for three cycles, which, unfortunately, was not successful. Her pain, which improved briefly after surgery, had recurred and was becoming intolerable. Although Clomid and IUI didn't work for Diane, several studies have shown that pregnancy rates with these methods are further enhanced after laparoscopic surgery. So, your fertility team may want to try this approach for three to six cycles to see if it works before trying in vitro fertilization.

Endometriosis and In Vitro Fertilization

To ease her symptoms from endometriosis, Diane underwent treatment with a GnRH agonist. After 3 months, her symptoms had significantly improved, so we followed with a cycle of in vitro fertilization. A single blastocyst-stage embryo (a 5-day-old embryo with about 60 cells) was transferred, and five other embryos were cryopreserved. Diane conceived and delivered a healthy child, Sarah, at term without complications.

In vitro fertilization, which will be explored in-depth in Chapter 12, represents the most successful means of overcoming endometriosis-related infertility, particularly in:

○ Women with more advanced endometriosis

○ Patients who have not conceived after surgical treatments or fertility drugs with IUI

○ Couples with compromised sperm

○ Women age 38 or older with mild or moderate endometriosis

Some studies have found that women with severe endometriosis have poorer egg production and therefore have a lower chance for pregnancy. It is possible that these women have undergone more extensive ovarian surgery, which may affect the ovarian blood supply and diminish the pool of available eggs.

There is some controversy about the best methods for dealing with an endometrioma prior to initiating an IVF cycle. If all other things are equal, the presence of a larger endometrioma appears to be associated with poorer responses to ovary-stimulating drugs and a lower number of eggs retrieved. Despite these facts, more recent studies have shown that overall pregnancy rates with IVF are not affected by the presence of an endometrioma.

The next question is whether it makes sense to operate on an endometrioma prior to an IVF cycle. The advantages are that doing so will improve access to normal ovarian tissue and eliminate the chance that the endometrioma will rupture during pregnancy. One disadvantage is that laparoscopy is an invasive procedure with associated risks, and there have been well-designed studies showing *no* improvement in pregnancy rates after surgery. Also, as previously mentioned, unless great care is taken to preserve normal ovarian tissue and blood supply, surgery may reduce the ovarian reserve.

It is important to note that if a woman has an *undiagnosed* solid ovarian mass, then this should be removed, a diagnosis made, and appropriate treatment undertaken (if necessary) before beginning any fertility therapy.

We often are asked whether laparoscopic surgery prior to an IVF cycle will improve pregnancy rates in women with endometriosis but without an ovarian

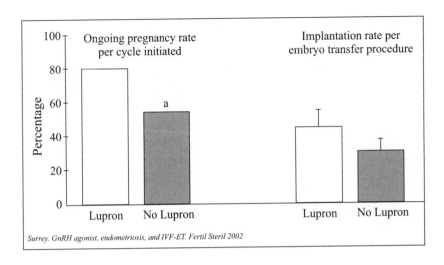

Figure 4: Effect of prolonged Lupron therapy on IVF outcomes in endometriosis patients

mass. We performed a study that showed the interval between surgical treatment of endometriosis and initiation of an IVF cycle had no effect on IVF pregnancy rates. Our finding has been confirmed by others.

As noted earlier, the medical treatment of endometriosis does not help spontaneous pregnancy rates. This may be because these medical therapies suppress ovulation, thus preventing pregnancy. Also, by the time the suppressive effect of these drugs has worn off, the negative effect of endometriosis on fertility may have recurred. The only way to avoid this problem is for the woman to conceive while her disease is suppressed, which is only possible with IVF.

We demonstrated this to be true in a randomized trial of 51 endometriosis patients who planned to undergo IVF. To suppress the symptoms of endometriosis, we gave patients a long-acting preparation of Depot Lupron (GnRH agonist leuprolide acetate) for several months prior to an IVF cycle. The result was significantly higher clinical pregnancy rates—78.3 percent versus 56.5 percent—than in a similar group of endometriosis patients who did not receive this agent (see Figure 4). Lupron works by lowering estrogen, which suppresses endometriosis. With endometriosis suppressed, the uterine environment is more receptive to the embryo.

Two other randomized trials from other centers have confirmed these findings.

Looking Beyond Endometriosis

Women with endometriosis often suffer chronic and acute pain as well as infertility. A careful evaluation of other factors causing infertility is critical prior to initiating therapy. Don't make the mistake of simply assuming that endometriosis is the only cause of your infertility.

Once you have nailed down endometriosis as a contributing cause of your infertility, there are several approaches to overcoming infertility. Some have proven more successful than others. Although IVF is clearly the most successful approach, other options may be appropriate for your situation (see "Options for Therapy for Endometriosis and Infertility," on this page). It is critical that you and your physician review all alternatives to select the correct approach that fits your needs, comfort level, and medical condition. This is a challenging diagnosis, but there is hope.

CHAPTER SIX

Tubal and Uterine Challenges

MARIE, 39, HAS two healthy children, ages 12 and 14, who were conceived without difficulty. A tubal ligation was performed after the delivery of her second child. Marie subsequently divorced and then remarried. Her second husband, Jack, 38, had not been married previously. Marie and Jack wanted to have a child together, so Marie came to our clinic to see if we could reverse her tubal ligation.

Marie's situation is not unusual. It's also fairly common for women to experience "sterilization regret" and decide they want to have more children, even if their marital status hasn't changed. Women in such cases must decide between two options: to surgically reverse the tubal ligation (tubal re-anastamosis), or to bypass the fallopian tubes entirely with in vitro fertilization (IVF).

Patient preference, maternal age, and the results of the fertility evaluation are all major factors in this decision. It is critical that a thorough evaluation, including ultrasound examination, ovarian reserve testing, and sperm function testing, be performed before a woman chooses to have her tubal ligation surgically reversed. For many patients, such as older women, women with borderline ovarian reserve, and couples with evidence of compromised sperm function parameters, another option, such as IVF, might be best. Surgical reversal is an ideal option for younger women with normal ovarian reserve whose partners' sperm function testing is normal.

Tubal Ligation Reversal Procedure

Typically, this procedure is performed under general anesthesia by making a small abdominal incision along the pubic hair line. Using an operating microscope and meticulous microsurgical techniques, the clips, rings, or scarred edges of the occluded tubes are removed. Once healthy tissue is identified, the tube is sewn back together using tiny sutures that are typically the width of a hair. Before completing the procedure, the surgeon confirms that the tube has been opened by injecting dye through a catheter placed into the uterus via the cervix.

A couple can typically attempt conception the month after surgery. If conception has not occurred within 6 months' time, an HSG (hysterosalpingogram) x-ray test can be performed to determine whether the tubes are functioning. In this test, a catheter is placed inside the uterus through the cervix and dye is injected to see if the tubes remain open. It is possible for scarring at the surgical site to cause adhesions or tubal reocclusion. If this occurs, IVF is typically recommended, because a second attempt at repairing the tubes is rarely successful.

Studies have shown that cumulative pregnancy rates range from 40 percent to 80 percent after a reversal procedure. However, the likelihood of conceiving in a given month ranges from 8 percent to 10 percent, which is considerably lower than the monthly rate achieved with IVF. Monthly conception rates are just that—the chance of pregnancy with 1 month of treatment. Cumulative rates are success over many months of treatment, such as a course of 6 inseminations over 6 months. Since IVF is done in 1 month, it is important to compare it to 1 month of other treatment.

The risk of ectopic (tubal) pregnancy is generally fairly low after these procedures given that in most circumstances, the remainder of the tube is normal in appearance and function.

The technique used in the initial sterilization plays an important role in whether reversal succeeds. The tubes are either cauterized, or closed with rings or clips. Pregnancy rates for reversal performed after tubal ligation employing cauterization, which causes greater tubal damage, are shown to be lower in several studies than when rings or clips have been applied.

If the tube is damaged in areas other than one site, then success rates are significantly compromised as well. Thus, it is critical to provide a copy of the operative and pathology reports from the initial sterilization procedure to your physician so that you get the best advice. The operative report tells your doctor how much of the tube was destroyed during the initial surgery and therefore how much is left to work with. There must be enough healthy tissue left for the tube to function properly. If, after surgery, the repaired tube is less than 4 centimeters long, then it is less likely to pick up the egg.

Although published reports about surgical procedures can give you a general sense of how likely it is that the surgery will succeed, the most critical factor is the skill and experience of the individual surgeon. You should feel free to ask your surgeon how many times he or she has done the procedure, or you can make inquiries about his or her reputation by asking other patients or nurses and by checking resources online. Personal references are the best.

To sum it all up, your choice between surgical reversal or in vitro fertilization should be based on the results of a complete fertility evaluation along with maternal age, the type of sterilization procedure performed originally, and your personal preference. It is critical that you and your physician thoroughly discuss the pros and cons of both approaches—both in general, and specifically in your case. Make sure that you also have an understanding of how successful your physician and clinic have been with both procedures.

The Solution for Marie and Jack

Marie and Jack consulted with a reproductive endocrinologist. As part of the evaluation, Marie's cycle day 3 level of follicle-stimulating hormone (FSH) was noted to be 9.8 international units per milliliter, near the upper limit of normal. Her follicle count was 6, and Jack's semen analysis was remarkable for a normal sperm concentration (34 million per cubic centimeter), but only 25 percent were motile and only 1 percent were normal. An FSH level of 9.8 (less than 10 is normal) means egg quality is borderline. (Less than 10 is normal.) Marie's follicle count of 6 means her supply of eggs is decreasing. A normal count is 13.

As a result of these findings, the couple elected to proceed with in vitro fertilization as opposed to reversing the tubal ligation. During the procedure, only

6 eggs were retrieved. Three were fertilized after intracytoplasmic sperm injection (ICSI) was performed, and the resulting embryos were transferred into Marie's uterus. One was brought to term and Marie delivered a healthy child, Josh, without complication.

Dealing with Tubal Blockage: Hydrosalpinx

Eileen, 35, had been trying to conceive for a year with her husband, Mark, 39. Both were in great health, and neither had been married before or had any history with pregnancies. Neither had undergone any significant surgeries. However, during her interview, Eileen said that while in college she had been diagnosed with chlamydia. She was treated with oral antibiotics and her symptoms rapidly resolved.

The couple first consulted Eileen's OB-GYN, who performed an initial evaluation, including baseline hormone levels, semen analysis, ultrasound examination, and an x-ray examination of Eileen's uterus and fallopian tubes (*hysterosalpingogram*, or HSG). The evaluation was normal with the exception of the HSG exam, which revealed that both fallopian tubes were blocked at the far end and dilated by a buildup of fluid, a condition called a hydrosalpinx. (The plural is *hydrosalpinges*.) The HSG exam is the traditional means of diagnosing tubal disease. For this x-ray exam, a small balloon-tipped catheter is placed in the uterine cavity through the cervix. Dye is then injected and a series of x-ray images are taken. Ideally, the dye should fill then spill through both tubes into the abdominal cavity, from which it is absorbed and excreted in the urine (see Figure 1).

The procedure is typically performed between the sixth and tenth day of a cycle to avoid the potential for exposing an embryo to radiation and to avoid menses. A course of oral antibiotics should accompany the procedure.

Tubal patency tests such as the HSG allow your doctor to look deep inside for any tubal obstruction or irregularity in the cavity of the uterus. (*Patency* refers to whether the tube is unobstructed.) A large study evaluated the HSG's accuracy in more than 4,100 procedures and reported a sensitivity of 65 percent for tubal patency in comparison with laparoscopy, another type of

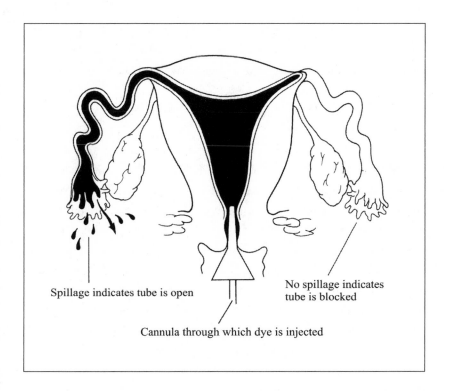

Spillage indicates tube is open

No spillage indicates tube is blocked

Cannula through which dye is injected

Figure 1: Hysterosalpingogram (HSG) exam

tubal patency test. This means that the HSG is correct in predicting tubes are open 65 percent of the time. So the HSG is not a perfect test, but is certainly very helpful. Laparoscopy, a "key hole" surgery performed through small incisions, remains the best method for diagnosing tubal abnormalities, but it is a much more invasive procedure than HSG and is usually considered only after an HSG has been performed.

Eileen's HSG found evidence of blockage at the *fimbriated* end of the tube. This is the end of the tube that picks up the egg at the time of ovulation. The fimbriae, the fringelike tissue at the edge of the fallopian tubes, are extremely delicate and can stick together as a result of infection, inflammation, even the presence of blood, or manipulation during surgery.

If the ends sticking together close off the tube, fluid can collect and cause a progressive dilation, causing a hydrosalpinx. The accumulation of this fluid damages the delicate cells that line the inside of the tube, making it more difficult for the tube to transport an embryo to the uterus even if the tube can be opened. Women with hydrosalpinges are also susceptible to ectopic (tubal) pregnancies.

This kind of tubal blockage is often caused by prior damage from sexually transmitted diseases such as gonorrhea or chlamydia, the latter of which may occur without any symptoms. (Symptoms that typically accompany chlamydia are pelvic pain, fever, or abnormal discharge.) Endometriosis can result in scarring and tubal blockage as well. Other causes include a prior ectopic pregnancy, abdominal infection (such as previously ruptured appendix), and prior pelvic surgery. It is important to note that use of IUDs has not been shown to cause tubal damage.

What is the best way to treat this type of blockage? Once again, it is critical to complete a full fertility evaluation prior to making a plan for therapy. If the couple is also found to have compromised sperm function or a low ovarian reserve, for example, IVF would be a more appropriate option than a complicated surgical procedure to repair the fallopian tubes.

In the past, surgeons had to treat blocked fallopian tubes using microsurgical techniques through an abdominal incision (*laparotomy*). Advances in minimally invasive surgical techniques now allow surgeons to perform those procedures through the laparoscope, employing lasers or fine scissors and sutures to open and repair the tubes.

Success rates with laparoscopic surgery vary based on the extent of tubal disease and the skill and experience of the surgeon. Unfortunately, the extent of tubal damage and of surrounding scar tissue cannot be accurately predicted by HSG, so laparoscopy may be necessary to determine whether the tubes can be repaired at all.

Pregnancy rates among women who have had their tubes surgically repaired vary. Generally speaking, success depends on how severely damaged the tubes were to begin with. Among patients with severely damaged tubes, pregnancy rates are generally less than 15 percent after surgery. Among patients with mild disease, surgical reconstruction may result in pregnancy rates high as 40 to 59 percent. However, the success rates with tubal surgeries are significantly lower than those achieved with IVF.

You should ask your doctor about the risks associated with these surgeries. The incidence of ectopic pregnancy after surgical repair ranges from 4 to 10 percent, which is 2 to 3 times higher than for the general population. Tubes that are repaired may still have scarring inside, causing an embryo to get stuck. There is also a chance that the tubes may reclose after surgery.

Yet recent studies have shown that even if a woman with a hydrosalpinx elects to proceed directly to IVF, surgery may still be necessary for her to conceive. Women with hydrosalpinges had significantly lower IVF pregnancy rates than women with other types of tubal blockage or normal tubes. Studies suggest that the inflammatory tubal fluid that drains into the uterus can be toxic to the embryo.

It would be logical to assume that stopping the flow of this fluid would reverse the negative effects on embryo development and implantation. Indeed, several well-designed studies have shown that removing damaged tubes (in a procedure called a salpingectomy) significant increases IVF pregnancy rates (see Figure 2).

Our research and that of others also has shown that closing off and cutting the tube with a hydrosalpinx at the uterine end of the tube yields beneficial results similar to removing the tube. Some have proposed a less invasive alternative to surgery for hydrosalpinges. This procedure would involve draining the harmful fluid with a needle guided by ultrasound at the time of egg retrieval for in vitro fertilization. But that method has not been consistently shown to be of benefit.

It is critical to have a frank discussion with your fertility specialist concerning the relative success rates and risks in your specific case of surgically repairing

Retrospective Series of 238 Cycles in 160 Patients

	Hydrosalpinx (%)	Tubal Factor No Hydrosalpinx (%)	Tubal Factor Corrected Hydrosalpinx	
			Post Failed IVF (%)	Prior to IVF (%)
Implantation/transfer	2.8	15.7	16.1	21.8
CPR/transfer	8.5	38.6	37.5	51.7

Figure 2: Surgical correction of hydrosalpinges and IVF

your fallopian tubes versus using in vitro fertilization, so that you can make an informed decision. Even if you have already decided to undergo a tubal reconstruction procedure, it is important to discuss the possibility of removing or closing an irreparably damaged tube at the same time so you can possibly avoid a second surgery if you end up trying in vitro fertilization again.

Eileen and Mark's Solution

Eileen and Mark consulted a reproductive endocrinologist at our clinic who also specialized in reconstructive surgery. Eileen underwent laparoscopy and was found to have massively dilated fallopian tubes on both sides with extensive scar tissue in the surrounding area. After a thorough dissection, the surgeon found that the ends of the tubes were completely abnormal. Both tubes were removed in an outpatient procedure.

But that was not the end of the story by any means. Eileen did not give up on her desire to have children, and neither did we. She underwent in vitro fertilization during the next cycle, and because the toxic effects of her hydrosalpinges had been eliminated, she was able to conceive. Thanks to the wonders of reproductive medicine, she later delivered healthy twin boys, Max and Adam, by cesarean section.

It wasn't so many years ago that Eileen and Mark might not have been able to have children of their own, but reproductive science has come a long way, and it continues to develop rapidly. It is important for patients to be informed about the latest methods and to take full advantage of every opportunity.

A few critical things to remember when considering tubal surgery:

○ Agree to a full fertility evaluation including an assessment of ovarian reserve and sperm function before making a decision of whether to undergo tubal reconstruction or IVF. This can save you time, money, and emotional anguish down the road.

○ A hysterosalpingogram, an x-ray exam of the uterus and fallopian tubes, is the standard means of evaluating the fallopian tubes, but is not as accurate as laparoscopy.

○ Reversal of tubal ligation can be highly successful in appropriately selected patients.

○ Despite the development of less invasive techniques, surgical repair of a hydrosalpinx results in generally low pregnancy rates except in the case of extremely mild disease.

○ You should give strong consideration to removing or permanently closing a tube with a hydrosalpinx blockage prior to in vitro fertilization in order to optimize your chances for pregnancy.

○ When comparing pregnancy rates between surgical repair of damaged tubes and in vitro fertilization, make sure to consider the specific outcomes achieved by the surgeon and IVF program you have selected. Some are better than others.

Dealing with Uterine Fibroids

Rachel, 38, and her husband, Sam, 41, tried to start a family for 2½ years without success. Sam had never been involved in a pregnancy before. Rachel had conceived during her college years, but elected to terminate the pregnancy, and that procedure had been performed without complication.

This couple was in good health, but Rachel told us she'd been having increasingly heavy periods for 4 years, to the point that she was using multiple tampons a day. In addition, she intermittently had midcycle bleeding, which was occasionally heavy, but only lasted for a day or two.

They consulted a reproductive endocrinologist, who performed an evaluation. Everything was normal except for the ultrasound examination, which suggested that Rachel had a "shadow" within the uterine cavity. In addition, the ultrasound found a small fibroid (measuring 2 centimeters) in the wall of her uterus, but it was not distorting the uterine cavity.

Rachel's case illustrates the importance of resolving any underlying medical or gynecologic problems before initiating treatment for infertility. Midcycle uterine bleeding may be caused by a benign structural problem such as a uterine fibroid or polyp, hormonal imbalances, uterine infection, or abnormal uterine cell growth.

Traditional techniques such as performing a baseline ultrasound examination or a hysterosalpingogram (HSG) may suggest abnormalities, but these methods are not particularly sensitive. A more accurate approach is a diagnostic *hysteroscopy*, an office-based procedure in which a narrow instrument bearing a tiny camera is gently placed through the cervix into the uterine cavity. Either carbon dioxide or a saline solution is used to open the uterine cavity so it can be viewed and any problems diagnosed. If necessary, a directed biopsy can also be performed. This procedure takes just a few minutes and requires only local anesthetic.

Another diagnostic approach is *sonohysterography*, a procedure which enhances the image obtained with traditional transvaginal ultrasound exams by simultaneously infusing the uterine cavity with fluid introduced through a small catheter placed in the cervix. If a patient has abnormal bleeding, a targeted biopsy of the uterine lining should be performed at the same time, particularly in women over age 30. Some studies have raised

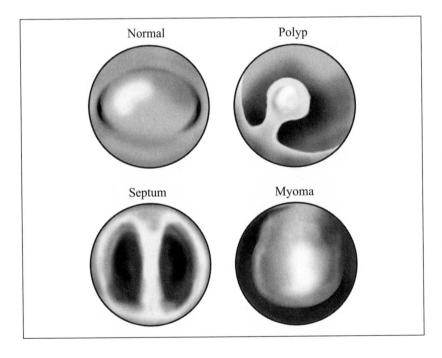

Figure 3: Hysteroscopic findings of normal and abnormal uteri

concern that in a patient with undiagnosed abnormal bleeding, this procedure could force abnormal cells through the fallopian tubes and into the abdominal cavity, but this risk has not been conclusively demonstrated.

It is very important to thoroughly evaluate the uterine cavity prior to in vitro fertilization even for women who have no abnormal bleeding. One study showed a very high incidence of uterine cavity abnormalities when hysteroscopy was performed after a failed IVF cycle. Even women whose HSG results are normal should consider having hysteroscopy. Even when the HSG indicates that the tubes are open, a hysteroscopy may show a problem in the uterus that the HSG did not show. An earlier study of IVF candidates who had previously had a normal HSG exam showed that pregnancy rates were decreased by two-thirds in those patients with abnormal findings with hysteroscopy.

The most common problems discovered with hysteroscopy are fibroids, polyps (usually benign overgrowths of glandular cells), scar tissue, and congenital abnormalities, many of which can be surgically repaired (see Figure 3).

As we noted, Rachel was found to have a uterine fibroid. Fibroids (or *leiomyomas*) are very common benign, smooth muscle tumors. They appear to have a racial predilection, being more common in black women and least common in Asian women. Many cause no symptoms at all. Others can cause pressure symptoms and abnormal bleeding, and may increase the likelihood of infertility and miscarriage. Pressure symptoms occur as the tumors increase in size. They start pushing on the surrounding organs such as the bowel and bladder, creating a feeling of fullness or pressure.

Fibroids are characterized by their location within the uterus: inside the uterine cavity (*submucosal*), inside the wall of the uterus (*intramural*), outside the wall of the uterus (*subserosal*), and on a stalk connected to the uterus (*pedunculated*) (see Figure 4). Fibroids inside the uterine cavity (submucosal) have been shown clearly to have a negative effect on IVF outcomes. They also increase the risk of miscarriage and are associated with an increased incidence of abnormal bleeding. Fibroids inside the wall of the uterus (intramural) that distort the uterine cavity may also have this effect. Other types of fibroids may cause symptoms, but do not appear to affect fertility or embryo implantation.

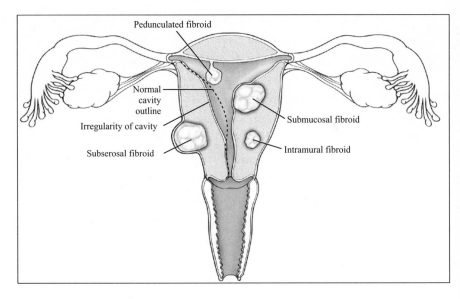

Figure 4: Types of uterine fibroids

Fibroids inside the uterine cavity are typically removed during an outpatient surgical procedure. The patient is put under an intravenous anesthetic, the cervix is dilated, and a wider hysteroscope is introduced into the uterine cavity. A wire loop (called a *resectoscope*) with an energy source is introduced through the hysteroscopy, which allows the surgeon to shave the fibroid and remove the tissue through the cervix.

Fibroids inside the wall of the uterus (intramural) usually cannot be removed completely in this fashion. They require an abdominal approach employing an incision in the uterus, fibroid removal, and subsequent uterine repair. This can be performed either through a small abdominal incision (mini-laparotomy) or, in certain circumstances, through a laparoscope.

For pregnant women who have undergone this procedure, cesarean section is usually the best option for delivery to minimize the risk of uterine rupture. Any surgery that involves an incision in the uterus is likely to weaken the uterine wall. Newer radiologic techniques for treating fibroids, such as uterine artery embolization and magnetic-resonance-guided ultrasound ablation, have

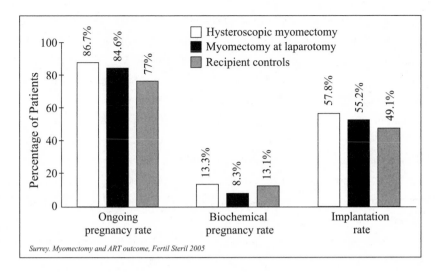

Figure 5: Cycle outcomes of oocyte donation

not yet been shown to be appropriate for women who wish to conceive, as they may damage the uterus.

Fibroids that affect fertility can be treated quite effectively. In a recent study at our clinic, we reported that ongoing pregnancy rates in women undergoing in vitro fertilization or egg donation cycles after removal of submucosal fibroids or intramural fibroids that were distorting the uterine cavity were the same as those in women who had no fibroids at all (see Figure 5).

Clearly, the uterine cavity should be thoroughly evaluated prior to in vitro fertilization and abnormalities should be treated, if appropriate. The mere presence of a fibroid does not mean that it is the cause of infertility or that it should be removed. However, those that do compromise fertility should be dealt with quickly; if they are, chances are excellent for a successful pregnancy.

The Solution for Rachel and Sam

Given his findings from the baseline ultrasound examination, Rachel's physician performed a hysteroscopic examination in the office. He had already found a

2-centimeter fibroid in the wall of Rachel's uterus. In addition, the "shadow" he had seen during her ultrasound turned out to be a 1.8-centimeter uterine fibroid inside the uterus (submucosal) taking up approximately one-third of the uterine cavity. Because of Rachel's age and her abnormal bleeding, the physician also performed an endometrial biopsy, the results of which were benign.

Rachel underwent an outpatient operative hysteroscopy procedure to remove the fibroid within the uterine cavity through the cervix, without the need for any incisions. Prior to surgery, the surgeon advised Rachel not to have the other fibroid removed because he felt that it was not causing her bleeding or her infertility. Her surgeon said the second fibroid would require a more extensive and invasive procedure for removal.

Rachel recovered well from her hysteroscopy. One month after surgery, she underwent a follow-up office hysteroscopy that revealed a completely normal uterine cavity with no evidence of a residual fibroid or scarring. That gave Rachel and Sam the all-clear sign to start their family. Nature did the rest. She conceived spontaneously 3 months later and delivered a healthy daughter at term.

Uterine Causes of Miscarriage

Ellen, 29, had been trying for nearly a year to have a child with her husband, Matt, 29. Both of them were in good health, but Ellen had experienced three first-trimester miscarriages. Her obstetrician had detected heartbeats for the last two fetuses on ultrasound examinations, but, in both cases, no heart beats were detectable a week later.

Ellen underwent a D&C for each of the last two pregnancies. The tissue from her most recent miscarriage was sent to the laboratory for genetic analysis and the embryo was found to be a normal male. The couple was referred to a specialist, who performed a standard evaluation for recurrent miscarriage. Everything was normal except for an ultrasound that suggested Ellen might have a uterine septum, a congenital malformation where the uterine cavity is partitioned by a longitudinal wall.

Repeated pregnancy loss can devastate a couple trying to start a family. Miscarriage occurs in approximately 15 percent of documented pregnancies, and that rate increases with maternal age. Repeated pregnancy loss, which is defined as three or more consecutive losses before 20 weeks of pregnancy, occurs in 1 to 2 percent of couples.

If you have had repeated pregnancy losses, your physician should try to assess whether the cause is genetic, hormonal, hematologic, or structural. In this section we will specifically address uterine abnormalities which can cause miscarriage. Miscarriages and repeated pregnancy loss are covered in depth in Chapter 8.

Congenital uterine anomalies are a common cause of recurrent pregnancy loss. They consist of alterations in the structure or shape of the uterus. The normal triangular shape of the inside of the uterus may instead look like a Y, or a banana, or may have a wall down the middle (septum), as was suspected in Ellen's case. These strange changes in structure occur early in fetal development, when the reproductive organs are forming.

Anomalies may occur at any time in this process. They range from a complete absence of these structures, to a single half of the uterus (unicornuate), to the formation of a wall between the two ducts within the uterus (septum) (see Figure 6).

The cause of these abnormalities is not known. However, one known cause is exposure of the fetus to DES (diethylstilbestrol), a compound administered in the late 1950s and early 1960s to prevent pre-term labor. DES causes a host of related abnormalities, most common among them a T-shaped uterus, which makes women susceptible to miscarriages.

Diagnosis of these disorders can only rarely be made accurately by routine ultrasound exam. Other methods of diagnosis are office hysteroscopy, three-dimensional ultrasound exams, hysterosalpingogram (x-rays known as HSG), magnetic resonance imaging (MRI), and sonohysterography, the method that infuses a fluid in the uterine cavity to improve the ultrasound image.

There is an association between mullerian defects (that is, defects in the uterus) and abnormalities in the kidneys and ureters (the tubes through which urine flows from the kidneys to bladder). Therefore, if a patient is found to have a significant congenital uterine structural abnormality, it is important that she

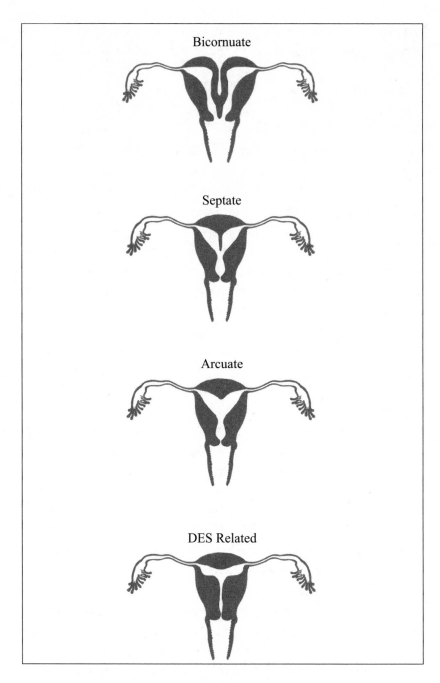

Figure 6: Uterine anomalies

undergo an imaging study of the kidneys and ureters to rule out an associated abnormality in the urinary system.

Treating Uterine Abnormalities

Some congenital uterine anomalies cannot be helped by surgery. The technical names for some of these abnormalities include *unicornuate* (in which there is a single half of the uterus), *didelphys* (in which there are two non-communicating cavities, usually with two cervices), or *bicornuate* (in which there are two separate but communicating cavities but one cervix). But fortunately, patients with these anomalies can still successfully carry a baby.

In contrast, a uterine septum can and should be surgically repaired. This procedure, known as *operative hysteroscopy*, can be performed on an outpatient basis. A thin telescope (a hysteroscope) is inserted through the cervix into the uterus. Fine scissors, a vaporization electrode, or a fiber laser can all be applied through the hysteroscope and used to remove the wall (septum) dividing the uterus into two halves. Once the septum is removed, the uterus has a normal triangular shape. This procedure is often performed under laparoscopic guidance to minimize the risk of uterine perforation.

Studies have shown that the incidence of miscarriage decreases from 88 percent to less than 20 percent after surgery to remove a uterine septum. Older techniques that require cutting out the septum through an abdominal incision have been largely abandoned.

Intrauterine *adhesions* (scar tissue) also can increase the risk of miscarriages and infertility. These adhesions can result from D&Cs or other surgeries inside of the uterus and can be repaired with operative hysteroscopy as well. If the adhesions are extensive, a balloon can be left in the uterus after the surgery for 1 week so that the scar tissue does not re-occur. Estrogen may also be used to help the uterine lining regenerate.

Women with severe uterine adhesions may also have a damaged uterine lining, which may block implantation or increase the risk of miscarriage. In this circumstance, it is possible that surgery will normalize the appearance but not the function of the uterus. This condition can be accessed by evaluating the thickness and pattern of the uterine lining with an ultrasound examination. Typically, a follow-up office hysteroscopy or saline sonohysterogram is performed several months after surgery to remove adhesions to confirm that healing is complete and that no adhesions remain or have reformed.

For the patient whose uterus cannot be adequately repaired, the best method to have a biological child is to select a gestational carrier, or, surrogate mother. This option is discussed thoroughly in Chapter 14.

The Solution for Ellen and Mark

Ellen underwent an office hysteroscopy, which confirmed the presence of a deep uterine septum extending three-quarters of the way down from the top (fundus) of the uterus. In addition, an MRI of her pelvis was performed to confirm that she had a uterine septum and not a bicornuate uterus. An ultrasound examination of the kidneys and ureters was also normal.

The description of all of this may sound ominous, but once the evaluation was completed and a diagnosis made, the solution was relatively easy for this patient and her husband. Ellen underwent an outpatient operative hysteroscopy in which her uterine septum was easily removed. Her surgeon decided to give Ellen an intrauterine balloon catheter to minimize the growth of scar tissue. In the follow-up office hysteroscopy performed 1 month later, her doctor found no evidence of a residual septum or scarring.

Four months later, Ellen conceived and went on to deliver a healthy child!

Key Points to Remember about Uterine Surgery

○ Any woman faced with infertility or recurrent pregnancy loss should be sure to get a uterine evaluation by office hysteroscopy or saline sonohysterography.

○ Uterine fibroids and larger polyps that distort the uterine cavity may inhibit implantation and should be removed. Fibroids which do not distort the cavity have not been clearly associated with infertility or recurrent pregnancy loss, and it is possible to have a healthy pregnancy without removing them.

○ The goal of surgically repairing the uterus is to use the least invasive surgery possible while leaving the uterus in the best condition possible to allow an embryo to implant.

○ If the uterine defect cannot be surgically repaired, the couple should consider using a gestational carrier.

CHAPTER SEVEN

Unexplained Infertility

SALLY ANN CAME to us with a diagnosis that drives many infertility patients mad, and I understand their frustration. She was only 32 years old, but she had been trying to conceive for more than 5 years. She'd taken what seemed like every infertility test known to science. Yet the only diagnosis her previous doctors could come up with was "unexplained infertility."

It's estimated that about 10 percent of infertility patients are given that diagnoses after their initial round of tests fails to show any explanation. A better term for unexplained infertility would be "unevaluated infertility." There is an explanation and a cause for every patient's infertility. A diagnosis of unexplained fertility just means that your doctor hasn't figured it out—yet.

So don't give up hope.

When women come to us with a diagnosis of unexplained infertility, the first two things we look at are the duration of their infertility and their age. Younger fertile women have approximately a 20 percent chance of spontaneous conception per month. In contrast, couples with unexplained infertility who are infertile for more than 3 years have spontaneous conception rates of 1 to 2 percent per month.

Human reproduction, compared with that of other creatures, is not very efficient. Mice and rabbits have almost 100 percent reproductive efficiency. Almost every time mice and rabbits are bred, they produce offspring. Humans are much more biologically and genetically complex; therefore, more things can go wrong and prevent reproduction.

Critical Factors Your Doctors Will Evaluate

As we've seen, for couples with unexplained fertility, the basic infertility workup often fails to evaluate or determine the cause. Our initial testing is a round of tests to check:

○ Sperm, including a semen analysis and test for antisperm antibodies

○ Cervical mucus to make sure the sperm can gain entrance into the uterine cavity

○ Uterus and fallopian tubes to confirm that the fallopian tubes are both open and that the uterine cavity is normal for implantation

○ Ovulation to confirm an egg is being released each month

○ Progesterone levels, as an indicator of the luteal phase

○ Follicle-stimulating hormone (FSH) and anti-mullerian hormone (AMH) levels, as rough indicators of egg quality (see Figure 1)

If all of these studies come back normal, we usually label the case "unexplained," but that does not mean we've thrown up our hands and given up. It

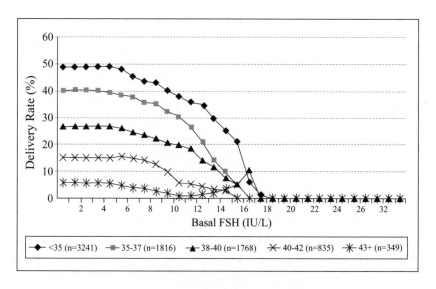

Figure 1: Predictive value of basal FSH in IVF delivery rates

just means that the cause of the patient's infertility was not determined in the first round of tests. There are many more tests we can do to try and answer the questions that remain.

Typically, we'll next look at whether the female patient's eggs travel from the ovary into the fallopian tube successfully, or whether something is interfering with their journey. With laparoscopic surgery, we can evaluate the pelvis for pelvic adhesions and endometriosis, both conditions that would keep the tubes from properly transporting the eggs.

Often in these cases, the patient may have had a history of chlamydia or some other type of pelvic infection. Or they may have used an IUD or had pelvic surgery, such as an appendectomy or removal of an ovarian cyst, which could also account for pelvic adhesions. Other patients with unexplained infertility may have a history of severe menstrual cramps or a family history of endometriosis. These are all conditions that your doctor can detect using laparoscopy, which is a reasonable next step in the evaluation.

If your doctor determines that the egg is in fact getting into the tube, the next question is whether it is getting fertilized. Some sperm that tests as normal still fails to penetrate or fertilize the female's eggs. There is no absolute way to know whether fertilization is occurring unless the patient gets pregnant on her own or we observe the fertilization directly during in vitro fertilization (IVF), when we add the sperm to the eggs in a Petri dish.

If the woman's eggs are entering the tube and being fertilized but she still does not conceive, the next step is to look at her embryos. Some couples have normal tests and their eggs fertilize readily but divide very slowly into poor-quality, fragmented embryos. The only way to know whether low-quality embryos are the cause of cause a couple's infertility is through in vitro fertilization.

When we do IVF with such patients, we usually allow half the sperm to penetrate the eggs naturally and perform intracytoplasmic sperm injection (ICSI) on the other half of the eggs. That way we don't have complete fertilization failure in the event that the first group of sperm fail to penetrate the eggs.

Couples who have poor embryo quality can often overcome this condition using in vitro fertilization. Sometimes we harvest 15 or more eggs, and 10 or more of these fertilize. When it comes time to transfer the embryo to the woman's uterus, all but one or two of the embryos will have developed very poorly and slowly and are not viable. Yet because the process started with so many eggs, the patients are able to create at least one healthy embryo for transfer, and they go on to have a successful pregnancy.

Abnormal chromosomes are another possible answer to unexplained infertility. To test for this problem, we do chromosome analysis, or *karyotype*. In this test we draw a tube of blood from both partners and check their 46 chromosomes. Some patients may carry a chromosomal abnormality that has no effect on them or their health but will cause their embryos to fail because of a chromosome imbalance. In such cases, the patient may have a history of miscarriages.

We will look also for a receptor called beta-3 integrin that some studies have found is necessary for implantation of the embryo. If the woman's eggs appear at first to be of normal quality, we still may go on and do a Clomid (clomiphene citrate) challenge test, which is a more complete and accurate method of measuring egg quality (described in Chapter 2).

In some cases, particularly with those patients who have had miscarriages, we may also test for antibodies known as *antiphospholipid* antibodies to be sure that the immune system isn't targeting the embryo itself as a foreign body or invader. We can also check the thyroid function as well as the prolactin level to rule out any hidden hormonal or endocrine causes of their infertility.

If we think a patient might have polycystic ovaries, we will also check levels of glucose, insulin, and other androgen or male hormones such as testosterone and DHEAS (dehydroepiandrosterone sulfate). We will also check levels of a hormone called 17-hydroxyprogesterone. Any disturbances in these hormone levels are treatable, and normalizing them may improve the patient's fertility.

These are just some of the tests that we can perform on patients with unexplained infertility to try to give them answers as well as a direction for their treatment. As you can see, much of what's called "unexplained infertility" is not really unexplained, but rather untested.

Unexplained infertility is simply a mystery awaiting a solution. If you are given this diagnosis, we recommend that you:

○ Seek a second opinion. Make sure to take your medical records, lab data, and x-rays with you.

○ Have your doctor repeat the semen analysis using the latest tests, such as the sperm DNA fragmentation test.

○ Request that your doctor do mycoplasma cultures for you and your partner, as some feel this infection can cause infertility. Mycoplasma are small bacteria-like organisms suspected of causing several urologic, obstetric, and gynecologic disorders, including pelvic inflammatory disease, urethritis, and pregnancy loss. Women whose reproductive tracts are colonized with mycoplasma can have higher rates of miscarriage. The organism lives in the male prostate gland and is transmitted during intercourse.

○ Even if your ovulation pattern is normal, discuss the option of intrauterine insemination (IUI) with washed sperm, combined with gonadotropin therapy to optimize your cycles (see Figure 2).

○ Ask your doctor to do an ultrasound after you ovulate to determine whether the follicle does in fact rupture and release the egg.

○ Suggest doing in vitro fertilization (IVF) to determine that fertilization is possible and to evaluate the egg quality (see Chapter 12).

○ Ask your doctor whether it is possible that you're having very early miscarriages before you get your period. Very early miscarriages can only be detected by measuring hCG in the blood just before or after a missed period. A positive pregnancy test followed by a fall of hCG to zero and the onset of a period means that a very early miscarriage has occurred. The causes include most of the same problems that lead to later miscarriages, such as genetic abnormalities of the embryo, luteal phase defects, uterine anomalies, etc.

Your doctor's job is to do the detective work to find the source of your infertility and then address it. As we've noted, the process of in vitro fertilization itself becomes the ultimate fertility test because it tells us about the quality of the eggs, the quality of the sperm, whether fertilization is occurring, and the quality of the embryo the patient is able to generate. Armed with all of this data, we can typically find a root cause for a couple's infertility.

In Sally Ann's case, we reviewed all of her tests and, indeed, they were completely normal. We explained that there appeared to be only two likely causes

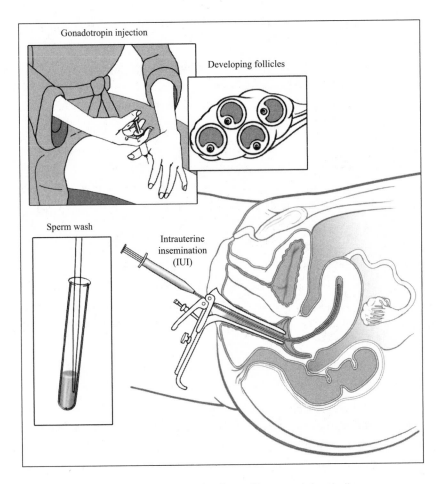

Figure 2: Intrauterine insemination with gonadotropin therapy

for her failure to conceive. One possibility was that her eggs were simply unable to access her fallopian tubes after leaving the ovaries. The second possibility was that her eggs were making it into the tube but failing to become fertilized.

Her husband's sperm had tested as excellent, so the latter possibility seemed unlikely. We concentrated on the possibility that Sally Ann's eggs could not make it into the fallopian tubes. I told her that there were two likely causes of this problem. The first was pelvic scar tissue or adhesions. The second was endometriosis. Sally Ann had no history of prior pelvic infection or prior surgery that would likely cause scar tissue, so we honed in on endometriosis.

Our first clue: Her sister and her mother both had endometriosis. Second clue: Sally Ann had experienced rather severe menstrual cramps since her teenage years. In light of those facts, we moved forward with diagnostic laparoscopy, in which a telescope attached to a camera is inserted through the belly button while the patient is asleep, allowing us to see all of the internal organs.

During Sally Ann's laparoscopy, we saw extensive endometriosis covering her ovaries and the pelvic sidewalls. Adhesions from the endometriosis also had caused her ovaries to stick to the back of the uterus, and her bowel was attached to the back of her cervix as well. Her disease was so extensive that only two-thirds of it could be removed laparoscopically. The remaining disease, on her bowel and other vital organs, made removal very dangerous.

We regrouped after her surgery and discussed our discovery that the eggs were indeed failing to travel from the ovary to the fallopian tube. In vitro fertilization was proposed as a way to bypass the fallopian tube trip. We moved forward with an IVF cycle the next month.

We are happy to report that Sally Ann—and her "unexplained infertility"—did very well with IVF, producing 15 eggs, 11 of which were fertilized, and 5 of which made excellent quality blastocysts on day 5. Two of these blastocysts were transferred, the other three frozen, and she conceived a twin pregnancy on her first IVF attempt!

We had to do some legwork, and extensive lab work, beyond the standard initial tests, but in a relatively brief time, Sally Ann's unexplained infertility was explained. In her case, laparoscopy was the critical procedure that revealed the hidden cause of her infertility and allowed us to move forward with the proper treatment.

Please keep in mind that unexplained fertility is simply a diagnosis commonly made after the initial round of tests does not turn up an obvious cause of infertility. It does not mean that your doctor is giving up. In fact, every year medical science comes up with new tools and methods for solving the mysteries of infertility.

CHAPTER EIGHT

Miscarriages

CHERYL HAD BEEN trying to have a baby but she suffered one miscarriage after another, enduring eight lost pregnancies in 8 years. By the time she came to our clinic, she felt like she'd been through hell and back. In our tests, we found that Cheryl had poor ovarian reserve—few eggs—but with the aid of medication and other treatments she was able to conceive a healthy son. Four years later, she had a second son without any help from us at all.

We love it when that happens!

Miscarriages are common, but that doesn't make them any easier on the women who suffer them. I speak nearly every day with women who've suffered multiple miscarriages, and I understand their emotional pain and their concern. In this chapter, I explain the causes of multiple miscarriages and the various treatments we pursue to overcome them.

Whether you have just one miscarriage or a series of them, the loss of a pregnancy is often traumatic, both physically and emotionally. Don't feel that you have to deal with this on your own. Emotional support is very important for women who've had even one miscarriage. Those who've suffered multiple miscarriages often have very high levels of anxiety and even depression.

Most infertility or OB-GYN clinics offer counselors or support groups for women suffering miscarriages. Online support groups also can be helpful. You can find information about online support groups at www.resolve.org or www.nationalshare.org.

While many women have just one miscarriage, the cruel reality is that every miscarriage you have increases your risk for another one. Miscarriage risk also increases as women age. The good news is that some of the latest research has found that after one or even two miscarriages, there is still as much as a 70 percent probability of having a successful pregnancy. After three, the chance of conceiving successfully is greater than 50 percent.

If you've read the previous chapters, you've already figured out that reproduction is not an efficient process. The more we learn at our clinic, the more we are convinced that it's a biological marvel to bring a healthy baby into the world without any hitches. There are so many things that can go wrong early in a pregnancy, and often they do.

Nearly 15 percent of all pregnancies result in miscarriage. A far greater number of conceptions (union of egg and sperm) end in miscarriage before a woman even realizes she is pregnant—as many as 50 to 70 percent.

Even though miscarriages are common, less than 5 percent of women will have two consecutive miscarriages, and only 1 percent or so will experience three or more. If a woman has three consecutive miscarriages, she then meets the criteria for "recurrent pregnancy loss."

If a patient has had two miscarriages, we initiate an evaluation to uncover a reason. In roughly half the cases, we are able to determine the cause of the miscarriages, which helps us determine how to help the patient sustain her pregnancies. Unfortunately, that still leaves us with 40 to 50 percent of those cases in which we can't figure out the cause.

Even among couples who have had more than five miscarriages, there is still a 50 percent chance that the next pregnancy will make it to term. This is very important to realize. Don't give up hope!

When we first meet with a woman who has had several miscarriages, we look at the most common factors, which include:

○ A family history of miscarriages

○ A family history of birth defects or chromosomal abnormalities

○ The age at which the patient's mother went through menopause (51 years is the average in the United States)

○ Whether she has had multiple D&Cs or uterine surgery

○ A history of thyroid dysfunction or diabetes

Genetic Causes of Miscarriages

Between 60 and 90 percent of miscarriages are thought to be caused by genetic factors. In these cases, something goes wrong during the first few cell divisions of an embryo. These miscarriages may be nature's way of preventing a pregnancy that is not proceeding normally. Much less common is the situation where either parent carries a genetic abnormality that is passed on to the fetus.

Approximately 5 percent of couples dealing with recurrent miscarriages may carry a genetic abnormality, the most common of which is called a *balanced translocation*. A balanced translocation occurs when part of one chromosome has switched places with a part of a different chromosome; for example, when part of chromosome 5 is attached to chromosome 10 and part of 10 is attached to 5 (see page 222). The parent does not typically have any hint that they are carrying this abnormality.

Yet if just one of these abnormal chromosomes gets passed on to the child, the child may have either an excess or deficient amount of DNA and this often results in a miscarriage. In rare cases, a child is born with this problem and faces significant medical problems.

It is important to realize that not all conception will be abnormal for couples with this problem. Even if either partner carries a balanced translocation, about 20 percent of the time, the embryo will be genetically normal. If you have a healthy child, it does not completely rule out the possibility that one of the parents carries this type of abnormality. The typical treatment for this condition is to go through in vitro fertilization with a preimplantation genetic diagnosis to genetically test the embryos before they are transferred into the uterine cavity. That way you can screen for the 20 percent or so that will be genetically normal and select those to transfer.

If you or your partner is found to carry a genetic abnormality, I recommend that you meet with a genetic counselor. That will give you a better idea of the percentage of embryos that might be affected as well as any other implications of your specific condition.

A genetic screening includes a blood test for a *karyotype*. Specific cells in the blood are grown, then they are tested to make certain that the proper amount of genetic material is present. This test does not screen for all genetic mutations—it screens simply for the proper number of chromosomes and the correct amount of DNA. It is important that both partners are tested because either partner can carry abnormalities. You will need to be patient, because it can take a month to get the results of this test.

Autoimmune Causes of Miscarriages

When miscarriages are caused by an autoimmune disorder, your body essentially rejects the developing embryo or fetus. The most commonly assessed autoimmune causes of miscarriages are lupus anticoagulant (LAC) antibodies and anticardiolin (ACL) antibodies. These antibodies are associated with blood clotting, and so it is suggested that anticlotting drugs may be helpful. In spite of the name, LAC antibodies can occur in people without lupus.

Women who have persistently elevated LAC, which interferes with blood clotting, or antiphospholipid antibodies, which cause blood clots, tend to have pregnancy problems, particularly miscarriages. Autoimmune issues are thought to be responsible for 3 to 15 percent of recurrent miscarriages. Treatment is typically heparin (a blood-thinner) and aspirin. Treatments that should be avoided are steroids and immunoglobulin therapy. Steroids taken during pregnancy can result in an increase in prematurity and diabetes. Another questionable course is immune therapy; it is expensive, has been associated with severe allergic reactions, and has no proven benefit.

Hormonal Causes of Miscarriages

Hormonal, or endocrine, problems can affect the development of an embryo. A very common endocrine abnormality in reproductive-age women is thyroid dysfunction. The thyroid is a specialized gland at the base of your neck that essentially controls your metabolism. A thyroid that is underactive (which is more common) or overactive (which is less common) can cause problems with pregnancy.

Blood tests that screen for thyroid abnormalities check for TSH (thyroid-stimulating hormone) or TSH and T4 (thyroxine). Thyroid abnormalities are fairly easy to correct, but it is very important for the patient to be meticulous about taking her thyroid medications.

A properly functioning thyroid gland in the mother has an important bearing on the brain development in the child. So this important not only in terms of miscarriage risk, but also in terms of fetal development.

If your thyroid gland is underactive and you are taking thyroid replacement, we encourage you to use only the name brand medications, not the generic. By law, generics can vary by as much as 20 percent, and in a medication that is administered in very low doses, we don't feel comfortable with that degree of variation. With most other fertility-related medications, such as Clomid, for example, generic substitutions are fine.

Another significant endocrine complication is diabetes. If you have diabetes and are trying to become pregnant, it is very important to optimize your glucose (sugar) control. The better controlled your glucose levels are, the less chance you will have for both miscarriage and risks of fetal anomalies. Your doctor can perform a blood test to determine your glycosylated hemoglobin (HbA1c) levels, which will show how well your glucose has been controlled. The American Diabetes Association recommends that pregnant women keep their HbA1c level below 7 percent. The higher above 7 percent you go, the higher the risk for birth defects and miscarriage. Some experts prefer an even lower number, such as 6 or 6.5 percent. Well-controlled diabetics do not appear to have an increased risk for miscarriage. If you have a family history of diabetes, had diabetes during a prior pregnancy, or are significantly overweight, ask your doctor to screen you for diabetes.

Another factor related to endocrine function is a woman's weight. We hear so much about weight loss and the obesity epidemic in the United States, it may sound redundant to encourage healthy lifestyles and weight control. Besides cardiovascular benefits and diabetes prevention, a normal BMI (body mass index) may help increase your chances for a healthy pregnancy.

We have known for a long time that among overweight women there are higher incidences of difficulty with labor, pre-eclampsia (complications related to high blood pressure), birth defects, cesarean section, and gestational diabetes.

Further, recent studies have shown women with a body mass index over 35 have twice the miscarriage rate of normal-weight women. (The National Heart Lung and Blood Institute provides a free BMI calculator at www.nhlbisupport.com/bmi/bmicalc.htm).

It's also worth noting that being underweight (that is, having a BMI under 18.5) has also been associated with poor reproductive outcomes. Being underweight contributes to low estrogen levels and poor progesterone production, both of which could increase the chance of miscarriage.

Anatomic Causes of Miscarriages

Structural problems with the uterus can lead to recurrent miscarriage (see also Chapter 6). One of the most troublesome is a uterine septum. This is an abnormal ridge of tissue that runs downs the middle of the uterus and is present there from the time a woman is born. Something occurs during the development of the uterus that leaves behind a band of tissue. Because it does not have a blood supply, this ridge is not a good place for the embryo to implant. If it does implant on the ridge, the embryo will result in an early miscarriage.

The key to this problem is making the correct diagnosis. Once the diagnosis is made, the treatment is pretty straightforward—you simply cut out that band of tissue, which can usually be accomplished vaginally during an outpatient surgical procedure. It is important to make certain that a uterine septum is not mistaken for a bicornuate uterus. The latter is a condition in which there are two separate uterine cavities. Your doctor can differentiate between the two conditions by sonogram, MRI, or laparoscopy. Unlike a uterine septum, a bicornuate uterus does not usually require surgery.

Other problems with the uterine cavity can include scarring inside the cavity or benign growths such as myomas (fibroids or leiomyomata) or polyps. If these are found inside the cavity, they are typically removed to normalize the cavity. Scarring may result from multiple D&C procedures, particularly those associated with the development of an infection. Sometimes, your doctors may not be able to pinpoint the cause of scarring. Some women with scarring will notice very light menstrual periods, and some women may have no periods, although many women will have no symptoms at all.

Fibroids are very common, as are polyps. With fibroids, the severity of the problem depends on where they are found. It's just like real estate—location, location, location! Fibroids in the wall or on the surface of the uterus often do not need any specific treatment and likely do not have any effect on a pregnancy, particularly if they are small.

Fibroids inside the uterine cavity are more problematic. Typically, we recommend removing them. This usually can be accomplished with a vaginal procedure done as outpatient surgery. Symptoms that may be associated with fibroids are heavy periods and pain during menstruation that may get worse over time; but again, women with fibroids may not have any symptoms at all.

The presence of a polyp is more of a judgment call. No one really knows what impact polyps have and whether large ones are more of a threat than smaller ones. We tend to be conservative, especially with patients who have had numerous miscarriages. We tend to remove all polyps to make sure the uterine cavity is a welcome home for babies.

Testing the Uterine Cavity

The best test for the uterine cavity is called a *hysteroscopy*. This is a test where you put a small camera—a *very* small camera on a very thin cable—inside the uterus and take a look. Hysteroscopy can be performed in the doctor's office or in an outpatient operating room. If it is performed in the office, a small flexible camera is typically used, and sterile water is placed in the cavity to separate the front and back walls of the uterus so the doctor can see well.

We typically perform this procedure between cycle days 6 and 10, and we recommend taking Motrin or Advil a few hours before. You may feel some mild to moderate menstrual-type cramps, but the procedure lasts typically for just a few minutes. Because you are awake, you can see on the camera monitor what your uterus looks like from the inside. Most women find this to be an interesting experience.

The advantage of doing this procedure in the office is that it does not require anesthesia and you can see the results in real time. The disadvantage is that you may feel some cramping, and if there is something that needs to be removed, it would then require a second procedure in the operating room. This is usually a same-day surgery done in the outpatient clinic.

Another test commonly employed to evaluate the uterine cavity is an x-ray test called a *hysterosalpingogram*, or HSG. This is performed in radiology and involves injecting a specialized dye, called a contrast, that shows up on x-ray. The contrast is injected into the uterus and fallopian tubes. The advantage of this test is that it will also tell you not only whether the uterine cavity appears normal, but also whether the fallopian tubes are open. The disadvantage to this test is that it may miss something small, such as a small polyp or fibroid.

This test also may cause some cramping, so taking Motrin or Advil a few hours before may be helpful. Also, if the radiologist warms up the contrast before injecting it, it may cause less cramping—so you might want to suggest to your radiologist or technician: "I take my contrast warm, please." If you are allergic to iodine, you are not a candidate for this test.

Recently, *sonohysterograms* are often being used for uterine cavity evaluations. This is a vaginal sonogram that instills water inside the uterus. By putting water inside the cavity, your doctor can visualize the uterus better than with a typical vaginal sonogram.

Blood-Clotting Disorders and Miscarriages

Thrombophilias are a group of disorders that make one prone to blood clots. If a pregnant woman has a tendency to form clots, it is possible that very small blood clots may form in the placenta and thereby compromise the blood flow to the embryo or developing baby. This is simply a theory, and there is lots of speculation and controversy as to whether thrombophilias really play a role in miscarriages. That being said, most reproductive endocrinologists will test for the most common inherited disorders, which include:

○ Antithrombin III

○ Protein S

- Protein C

- Factor V Leiden

- Prothrombin gene mutation

If your test comes back abnormal, but you don't have a clinical history of clotting problems—such as a blood clot in your legs or a pulmonary embolism—then it is a bit tricky to decide whether to treat for a clotting abnormality. If your physician decides to treat you, the most common treatment is to administer a blood thinner—such as lovenox, a low-molecular-weight heparin starting early in pregnancy.

Taking a blood thinner does carry risks—as it increases your tendency to bleed. For example, if you were in a car accident and you were on a blood thinner, your injuries could be much worse than if you were not on a blood thinner. We usually address this on a case-by-case basis because there is no one protocol that applies to all patients.

Luteal Phase Defect

Progesterone is a hormone produced in the ovaries, the placenta, and the adrenal glands. It helps prepare your body for conception and pregnancy and regulates the monthly menstrual cycle. The concept of a *luteal phase deficiency* was first proposed in 1949. The proposition was that some women's bodies do not make enough progesterone to maintain the pregnancy. And if the progesterone levels are too low, the pregnancy will either fail to implant or result in early miscarriage.

Many tests have been developed to try to determine whether a woman's progesterone production is sufficient. This includes measuring blood levels of progesterone or doing an endometrial biopsy—where the uterine lining is sampled to look for progesterone problems. It makes sense that this is an important issue for fertility and pregnancy. The problem is that so far the best studies on this issue have failed to find a link between luteal phase deficiency and infertility or recurrent miscarriage. And giving women supplemental progesterone has failed to show any benefit.

On the other hand, progesterone supplements are important for women undergoing in vitro fertilization. They do not ovulate and therefore may not form a normal *corpus luteum* (the structure that typically makes progesterone). They also may take medication that decreases their production of progesterone, so these women do need additional progesterone. Many clinics will still give women with multiple miscarriages supplemental progesterone, as the risks are quite low, but the benefit in non-IVF cycles is unproven.

Age Factors in Miscarriages

The chance for miscarriage increases as women get older; in fact, more than 50 percent of pregnancies in women above age 43 resulted in a miscarriage.

Because your eggs age with you, they become less healthy and more susceptible to genetic abnormalities. We think that is why miscarriage rates increase as women get older. Although there is no specific test that will tell you exactly how healthy your eggs are, some tests can give us information above and beyond that of age alone.

The most common is a test called an FSH (follicle-stimulating hormone) test. This is typically done on day 3 of your menstrual cycle and involves a blood test. A normal value is below 10 international units per milliliter. The higher the FSH, the worse the prognosis, because high FSH levels usually indicate poor egg production.

Another test for your eggs—also known as your "ovarian reserve"—is the Clomid challenge test (see also page 33), or CCCT. This test involves taking Clomid (the brand name of clomiphene citrate) days 5 through 9 of the cycle. We then compare a woman's FSH and estradiol levels before (on day 3 of cycle) and after (on day 10 of the cycle) she took the Clomid. The higher of the two FSH values is your result. This test is more predictive than just the day 3 FSH and therefore is used more often in women 35 years old or older, and on women who have had a poor response to fertility medication treatment.

FSH values do vary month to month, so if you were to check your FSH for 3 months in a row it is quite likely that you will get some variation among the values. Your prognosis is based on the highest value. Be warned that there is no validated treatment to lower your FSH values, nor is there any benefit to waiting to undergo treatment for a month when your FSH may be lower. There are some unscrupulous operators out there who claim they can reduce your FSH values. Do not believe them.

New tests being developed for ovarian reserve assessment look at inhibin B levels and anti-mullerian hormone (AMH) levels. Inhibin B is a protein hormone produced by your ovaries that inhibits FSH, which, in turn, helps your follicles develop. Levels of inhibin B decrease with age. AMH is also produced by the ovaries and reflects the number of follicles present. These tests are still under investigation and have not been as well validated as the FSH and Clomid challenge test.

Another fairly easy test is an *antral follicle count* (AFC). An AFC measures the number of small follicles in the ovary as seen by ultrasound. A typical number is greater than ten, and less than five is a cause for concern.

Emotional Aspects of Multiple Pregnancy Losses

Deb Levy

Deb Levy, one of our clinic's psychological counselors, has a lot to offer patients who've experienced multiple miscarriages, so we asked her to offer some guidance to our readers, too.

Women who have suffered multiple pregnancy losses may experience extreme symptoms of grieving. As discussed in the book *On Death and Dying*, by Dr. Elisabeth Kubler-Ross, grieving can include many different emotions, and patients who have suffered miscarriages often experience a wide range of feelings, including symptoms of depression and anxiety. These emotions may feel magnified after a miscarriage, so counseling can be beneficial.

It is not uncommon for those suffering multiple pregnancy losses to turn their anger, a normal aspect of grieving, upon themselves. They may blame themselves and wonder what they could have done to prevent the miscarriage.

It is not uncommon, either, to have patients who've suffered recurrent miscarriages say they feel guilt or shame. Often, women say, "I feel like a failure." Others may feel that they were unable to carry out one of the most basic "tasks of womanhood." So, they may find themselves feeling like less of a woman, less of a wife, or simply inadequate.

Patients and medical staff have noted that some of the terminology used by doctors and nurses doesn't help. When patients hear us talk of "failed IVF cycles" and "habitual aborters," they can't help but feel emotionally drained.

American culture hasn't come to terms with grieving and loss as well as other cultures. That is why many couples choose not to tell others of their pregnancies in the first trimester. They are hesitant to "disappoint" their friends or family members who might enthusiastically follow the pregnancy.

This reluctance to talk about early pregnancy is especially common among those who have suffered multiple pregnancy losses, as they don't want to go through the process of explaining the loss time and time again. There also may be the fear that others will blame or judge them.

All couples have a right to privacy, of course, but you don't want to get in a situation where you are alone with your grief, without the support of friends or family members and the perspective they can provide. The stress of grief and the feelings of guilt or shame can be too much for one person or even a couple to bear alone. It may be even dangerous to your emotional and physical health. So this is not something you want to go through alone. Understand that grief is a natural process and nothing to fear or be ashamed of, but if ever there is a time when you should lean on those closest to you for support, this is it.

We also have patients tell us that when they reach out to friends and family after losing a pregnancy, they sometimes get responses that, whether intentional or not, seem hurtful, insensitive, or less than supportive. The fact is the even those close to you may not know exactly what to say in such cases, and sometimes, they may not express themselves well. The same thing happens at funerals and wakes, when people sometimes say inappropriate things simply because they are at a loss for words at such an emotional time.

Those who have suffered multiple pregnancy losses also may experience symptoms associated with posttraumatic stress disorder. In these cases, the miscarriage may be replayed in one's head over and over so you feel as though you are constantly re-experiencing the trauma. As a result, you may feel depression or anxiety at high levels. Or, you may shut down emotionally so that you feel empty, or without hope. Typically, patients in that frame of mind say things like "I'm never going to have a baby."

Physical manifestations, such as insomnia, flashbacks, or nightmares, can also be apparent with posttraumatic stress. Following a loss, many patients also report a desire to get pregnant again, and sometimes this is coupled with a conflicting and very intense fear of getting pregnant again.

Patients who have suffered multiple pregnancy losses report significant emotional and physical stress, so counseling and group support are strongly recommended. There is no instant cure for the very natural process of grief, unfortunately. No counselor has the ability to simply make the emotional anguish go away, but counseling can help you understand your emotions as valid and normal.

It can also help you manage your grief if you memorialize or honor the loss with a ceremony or funeral. I also recommend support groups, where you can share your feelings and find others who have been through similar grief. Often, there is no better way to get through your grief than to see that so many others have gone through the grieving process and emerged from the experience as stronger people.

I counsel patients to practice good self-care through journaling, meditation, exercise, counseling, massage, or other coping tools. These can help you manage both the emotional and physical manifestations of loss.

Nothing can quickly remove emotional pain from the loss of a pregnancy, and as long as you understand that grief is a natural process, you can allow yourself to feel all the various emotions that may arise. You should not feel it necessary to force yourself to feel better or to hide or bury your emotions, because they will manifest themselves in other ways, even unpredictable ways. We've had patients who've stifled their grief only to find themselves breaking down in their cars or offices, or lashing out at loved ones or coworkers "for no reason."

It helps to know that while you may never forget the lost pregnancy, you can expect to accept it one day and then move on; one day you will again feel like your normal self.

CHAPTER NINE

Male Infertility

IT IS NOT unusual for couples to come to us thinking that *she* has a fertility problem only to discover instead that *he* has a problem. Studies have shown that 40 percent of infertility cases are related to male reproductive problems, which range from physical abnormalities and ejaculatory malfunctions to poor sperm production and immunological disorders. Around the globe over the past 50 years, sperm counts have gone down dramatically, according to the World Health Organization. So, this problem is not going away. Fortunately, we have made great gains in treating male infertility.

We tell couples that infertility is always a *we* problem. Neither partner in a couple is to blame. Yet, just as many of the women we treat often say they can't be a "real woman" until they have a child, men may see infertility as a challenge to their masculinity.

It is also true, however, that men often are not as driven as women to overcome their infertility, which can dismay their female partners. Some men feel that having children is "a woman's business." So they may disengage from the fertility struggle and not wish to pursue treatment as avidly as women.

Most people don't realize that it frequently takes both the male and female partner to resolve infertility issues. Infertility is not a female issue. It is not a male issue. It is a couple's issue, as our patients Dave and Sandra discovered.

Three years before coming to our clinic, Dave learned from another physician that his sperm count was zero and that the only option for him and Sandra to have children was to use donor sperm. This diagnosis was not well received, and Dave and Sandra were at odds over accepting donated sperm. Doing so would mean that the child would not carry Dave's genes.

Their relationship deteriorated and the couple separated. Happily, they reconciled 2 years later, and Dave came to us for treatment. This time, he and Sandra both were willing to consider donor sperm insemination. First, however, we asked Dave to undergo the standard workup of tests and examinations. We did blood work, a urology consultation, and ultrasound examinations.

Based on our findings, we concluded that Dave had a condition called *non-obstructive azoospermia*. Basically, this means that there were no sperm present in his ejaculate even though there was no blockage in the vas deferens detected. It appeared that Dave's testicles probably were making sperm, but not in enough quantity for them to make it all the way out the reproductive tract. His sperm were getting stuck like salmon that could not make it upstream to spawn.

Our team felt that Dave had a better option than going with a sperm donor. Instead, he could undergo a testicular sperm extraction procedure. His sperm could not get out, so we could go in after them. Dave was anesthetized so that we could do a small biopsy of the testicle to see if there were sperm present. We found just a few, but enough to accomplish our mission with in vitro fertilization.

Dave and Sandra were overjoyed when we told them there was a good chance they could have a child without using a sperm donor. They also were more than a little disturbed. Their marriage had nearly been destroyed and they'd lost nearly 3 years as parents because their first physician had not done a complete examination.

Some men with non-obstructive azoospermia have a chromosomal or genetic abnormality, so we checked Dave's blood to be sure his 46 chromosomes were all in order. We also checked to make sure that the so-called Y deletion, a missing part of the Y chromosome, was not present; if it had been, it might have been the cause of his infertility. These blood tests assured us upfront that we would be injecting genetically normal sperm into Sandra's eggs and that we would be creating the best circumstances possible for the couple to have a healthy baby.

Sandra was evaluated next and she was found to be a good candidate for

IVF. She was relatively young and she had a healthy uterus. We performed an ultrasound and tested her follicle-stimulating hormone (FSH) and anti-mullerian hormone (AMH) levels, all of which indicated she had plenty of healthy eggs available. On the same day that we retrieved Sandra's eggs, we went in after Dave's sperm. We then injected his sperm into his wife's eggs. Multiple embryos resulted, and two were transferred to Sandra's uterus.

Sandra conceived and 9 months later delivered a child without complications. Even better, this couple still has three embryos and some of Dave's sperm frozen, so they could have more children if they want to.

Finding the Source of Male Infertility

When couples come to us, our initial evaluation to find the source of their infertility always includes testing the male. Fortunately, men get a break here, as it is typically easier to test for their fertility problems than for women's. By performing a semen analysis, we can assess whether there is a problem present in the male. If we find one, the next goal is to identify the cause, and, if it is reversible, correct it.

We can help patients like Dave, with no sperm present in the ejaculate, conceive a child of their own with assisted reproductive techniques.

It may be possible for a patient who has significant abnormalities in his semen analysis to improve the quality of his semen sample so that in vitro fertilization (IVF) will no longer be necessary. Instead, intrauterine insemination (IUI), also known as artificial insemination, may be a reasonable option. And if a man has borderline quality and quantity of sperm, with intervention, it may be possible to upgrade him from intrauterine insemination procedures to natural conception. Although these interventions typically take time, they may lower the cost and the degree of invasiveness of treatment.

It is in the patient's interest to ask for the least invasive and most cost-effective treatment possible. In this era of escalating health care costs, your doctors have a responsibility to be aware of the economic repercussions of their recommendations and treatment. This is especially true in treating couples with infertility issues. They may have to pay out of pocket, because often health insurance does not cover the costs of diagnosis or treatment.

Your infertility team should also try to identify any potential genetic issues for the male and female before conception, as a significant genetic issue may influence a couple's ability to conceive, or it may affect their decision to proceed with assisted reproductive techniques.

Avoiding the Blame Game

Most of the time, the female partner initiates the infertility evaluation. Many men are reluctant to admit that they may be infertile. They may feel that such issues threaten their manhood. In fact, it is rare for a man to come in on his own for fertility testing.

We usually see the male partner only after the female goes to her gynecologist complaining of difficulty conceiving. Commonly, it is at that point that the gynecologist recommends that her husband have a semen analysis, either while she is being evaluated or afterward.

It's important for both partners to avoid the "blame game." Blaming one another can not only damage a relationship, but it can also lead to an inappropriate sense of guilt and inadequacy, and even to depression.

It has been estimated that nearly 50 percent of male infertility cases are *idiopathic*, meaning that doctors cannot identify the source of the problem. Fortunately, with the use of assisted reproductive techniques, it is still likely that even in those cases, the couples will successfully conceive and have a healthy child.

Great strides have been made in understanding the causes of male infertility and in the development of interventions to correct these issues. However, our understanding of male infertility at the most basic molecular level is still very much in its infancy. As medical scientists gain greater insight into issues with sperm DNA and into the molecular mechanisms of fertilization, they are likely to develop more drug interventions to assist conception. Scientists have identified some genetic issues associated with male infertility, and we've developed the ability to test for them, but it is likely that there are undiscovered genetic abnormalities that impede natural conception.

Your physician should do his or her best to help both the male and female partners feel comfortable and supported in their efforts to start a family. If your infertility doctor doesn't do this, you should find one who does. Being comfortable with your physician will allow you to be forthcoming and honest, which is absolutely critical for your successful treatment. It is important that you be able to accurately describe your sexual habits, success or failure to conceive with previous partners, history of sexually transmitted diseases, or history of drug use, because even though such topics might be embarrassing, all these factors may have some impact on your ability to father children.

I find that having both partners present at all the appointments facilitates communication and helps them understand the process. Most men willingly admit that they are not the greatest communicators, nor are they the best at relaying information to their partners. If the woman never attends the discussion sessions with the doctor, the man may not be able to fully pass on to his partner what is going on with him, what the treatment options are, and the complete list of advantages and disadvantages of each alternative.

I often make recommendations for the male partner that are dependent on the fertility status of his female partner. It would be ridiculous and futile, for example, to attempt to correct minor abnormalities in a male's semen analysis if his female partner in unable to conceive without IVF. Having her present at our discussion improves our understanding of her situation, and the "big picture" of how to best treat their infertility.

In the same manner, the man's presence at the woman's appointments will improve his understanding of her situation. Such knowledge will help couples make good decisions about the most efficient and cost-effective way to conceive. The involvement of both partners from the start of the evaluation will minimize the discord that often results from the emotional and financial strain of infertility.

Male Fertility Evaluations, Step by Step

The first step in evaluating the male is to get a thorough medical, social, developmental, reproductive, and sexual history. Although men's fertility typically lasts much longer in life than women's, the male's age is pertinent. The female partner's age is also important, as it may influence the urgency of evaluation and intervention, and may alter the recommendations for treatment.

If you are a man undergoing a fertility evaluation, your doctor will want to know whether you have ever fathered a child because that helps determine potential causes. *Primary infertility* occurs when a man has never been capable of fathering a child, while *secondary infertility* is an acquired condition that occurs after he has previously fathered a child. In the case of secondary infertility, a congenital or genetic source for the patient's problem can be ruled out. Similarly, if the female has conceived in the past with a prior partner, it suggests that the male partner may have fertility issues.

The doctor will look at your medical history to see if both of your testicles were in the scrotum at birth or if you had undescended testes. It is also important to know whether you had surgery to place the testicles into the scrotum. A history of undescended testes is associated with subsequent decrease in fertility.

Your doctor will also have a list of questions about your sex life, such as:

○ Did you have a normal puberty? If so, at what age?

○ When did you become sexually active?

○ How frequently do you and your partner engage in sexual intercourse? Is it timed around the female's ovulation?

○ Do you use lubricants? If so, what kind? (Some fairly innocuous-appearing lubricants, such as K-Y Jelly, can impede sperm motility and lower the chances of conception.)

○ Do you have any libido issues, erectile dysfunction, or ejaculatory problems? If so, how long have you had them?

○ How long has it been since you and your partner stopped using contraception? The implications of the evaluation are significantly different for a couple who has had unprotected intercourse for several years and a couple who has only just begun to try.

Again, taking a complete medical history is imperative in trying to solve the mystery of infertility for the male and female. Diabetes, neurological problems, cancer, autoimmune disorders, and cystic fibrosis are among the medical conditions that can affect male fertility. Prior surgeries on the groin or scrotum can obviously have an effect on a man's fertility, as can certain pelvic and abdominal surgeries such as hernia repair.

You should also tell your doctor about any medications you're taking, as there are several that can affect a man's fertility. One of the drugs that is the most detrimental to fertility is testosterone, which is sometimes given as a supplement or in the form of a variety of anabolic steroids sometimes abused by athletes and bodybuilders. Both testosterone and anabolic steroids can prevent normal stimulation of testicles by the pituitary gland, and lead to atrophy (or, shrinkage) of the testicles and a subsequent decrease in sperm production. The reversibility of this testicular atrophy and impairment in sperm production is in part dependent on the amount used and the duration. Other drugs that can affect sperm production and function include sulfasalazine, cimetidine, certain psychotropic medications, calcium channel blockers, cyclosporine, colchicine, and certain antibiotics. Infertile patients who require testosterone supplements to treat other conditions might benefit from altering their medication while they're trying to conceive. For example, it is typically possible to stimulate increased testosterone production from the testicles without impairing sperm production by using hCG (human chorionic gonadotropin).

Cytotoxic chemotherapy can profoundly affect sperm production. The agent used, the dose, and the duration of its use will determine to what degree sperm production will return after receiving chemotherapy. For this reason, patients who are facing chemotherapy are always encouraged to have their sperm frozen and stored in a sperm bank (cryopreserved) before they start this treatment.

Radiation therapy on the testicles can damage sperm production irreversibly. The germ cells within the testicles are notoriously sensitive to effects of radiation therapy. For this reason, it is important to shield the testicles to the greatest extent possible in order to minimize the effects on radiation. This is another situation in which a patient should consider banking his sperm prior to treatment.

Environmental and Social Factors
That Affect Male Fertility

Even Marlboro men know these days that smoking cigarettes is bad for their health, but often our male patients are surprised to learn that smoking affects their fertility. All smoke—whether from cigarettes, cigars, or marijuana—contains a multitude of toxic constituents that can impair sperm production. We recommend that men who want to have children discontinue smoking altogether.

Although alcohol in moderation has no significant detrimental effects on a man's fertility, in excess and on an ongoing basis, alcohol can alter the body's hormones and lead to changes in sperm production.

The testicles are packaged in the scrotum because they need to be a few degrees cooler than body temperature in order for sperm to develop normally. Any behavior which elevates scrotal temperature—spending a lot of time in a hot tub, Jacuzzi, steam room, or sauna; wearing tight-fitting underwear, or even using a laptop—may alter sperm production. Similarly, any illness with a fever, even a common cold, can transiently raise scrotal temperature and diminish sperm quantity and quality.

One common cause of elevated scrotal temperature is a *varicocele*, a group of dilated veins originating from the testicle. Varicoceles are relatively common, occurring in approximately 15 percent of adult men. Not all men with varicoceles have issues with infertility; still, a varicocele is the most common cause of correctable male infertility. The dilated veins act as a radiator and raise scrotal temperature, which can have a deleterious effect on sperm production. Fortunately, varicoceles can be surgically corrected, and in 50 to 60 percent of cases, the patient's semen analysis is significantly improved.

A man's general physical health is another important "environmental" factor in male fertility. A patient should expect his doctor to examine him for general appearance, including height, proportions of the body, presence of obesity, and the presence of prominent breast tissue. The doctor should also make a careful evaluation of the anatomy of the genitals as well. When examining the genitals, the doctor will assess the size of the penis to make sure it is within the normal range, and will check the size and location of the urethral opening as well. The size, location, and texture of the testicles will also be evaluated, as will the *epididymis*, the accessory gland coming off the back of the testicle and the location where sperm mature, and the *vas deferens*, the tubular structure that transports sperm from the scrotum, through the groin, and to the prostate, where it mixes with seminal secretions.

Lab Work for Male Infertility

It is fairly straightforward to assess whether there is a male infertility issue, but certainly it is more difficult to assess the source of the problem. The first step in the laboratory evaluation is to perform a semen analysis.

Although many laboratories perform semen analyses, specialized andrology labs should be used, because they are more experienced with semen analyses and are likely to provide more reliable results.

The patient is asked to abstain from ejaculation for at least 72 hours prior to the collection of a semen sample. Although patients may desire to collect the semen sample at home, it is preferable for them to collect a semen sample in the laboratory to ensure rapid evaluation of the sample. The patient is instructed to collect the semen sample by masturbation in order to lower the risk of incomplete collection and contamination from other body fluids. Complete collection of the sample into the container is important, as the sperm may not be equally dispersed through the entire ejaculate.

Once the semen sample is processed, the initial assessment is the semen volume. The sperm concentration, typically referred to as the count, is critical to know. Normal counts are typically greater than 20 million sperm per cubic centimeter. A count lower than this will make it more difficult to conceive. Sperm motility, or, the percentage of sperm swimming, is also assessed. The normal range is typically greater than 40 percent.

Finally, the lab assesses the sperm's morphology, meaning, what percentage of sperm look normal by very strict criteria. The normal measure is 4 percent or higher. Other aspects of the semen analysis evaluated include how viscous (thick) the sample is, the color of the sample, the pH, and whether white blood cells are present. If there is an abnormality in any of these variables, natural conception may be impaired.

It is very common to have some fluctuation in the sperm count, the motility, and morphology. For this reason, it is imperative to have at least two semen analyses performed on two separate days to fully assess male fertility.

Other laboratory tests may be called for, particularly if the sperm count is low, including an assessment of pituitary hormones LH (luteinizing hormone), FSH (follicle stimulating hormone), TSH (thyroid stimulating hormone), and prolactin. These tests can clarify whether the testicles are being adequately stimulated to make sperm. Checking serum testosterone levels and estradiol levels gives your doctors a handle on testicular function and hormone metabolism within the body. Hormone levels are easily checked by testing a blood sample. In addition, hormonal levels can frequently be manipulated with medications to further stimulate sperm production.

For patients like Dave, who have either no sperm in their ejaculate (azoospermia) or very low counts, it may be necessary to perform a genetic analysis. There are certain identifiable genetic defects that are associated with male infertility and can be detected with blood work. Checking the number and arrangement of the 46 chromosomes (using a test called a *karyotype*), checking a *Y-chromosome microdeletion* (a genetic issue associated with infertility), and assessing whether the patient is a carrier of cystic fibrosis are all important genetic tests that can help determine whether the patient has adequate sperm while also alerting the couple to any risk of passing on certain abnormalities to their offspring.

Abnormal Semen and Its Impact on Fertility

Having an abnormal semen analysis does not mean that one cannot father a child. Once again, the physician's goal is to identify reversible causes of the semen analysis and correct them so that the patient can conceive with the least amount of intervention and at the lowest cost possible. Improvements in the semen analysis do not occur overnight. Because each generation of sperm takes an average of 72 days to develop, any intervention will take at least that long. For this reason, typically a repeat semen analysis will not be performed sooner than 3 months after an intervention.

If the semen analysis cannot be improved, then some form of assisted reproductive technique will be necessary. If the semen analysis is only mild to moderately abnormal, then intrauterine insemination (IUI) is a reasonable option, assuming the female partner is a good candidate for this method. IUI is a procedure which involves collecting a semen sample, processing it, and injecting it via a small catheter through the female partner's cervix into the uterus at the time of her ovulation. This procedure is relatively noninvasive and relatively inexpensive.

Because in vitro fertilization (IVF) requires only a few sperm rather than millions, it can be extremely useful for the individual with an abnormal semen analysis. IVF has allowed men like Dave father a child when they would otherwise be unable to have their own biological child.

The Absence of Sperm and Fertility

Men undergoing treatment for infertility are often told, as Dave was at the beginning of this chapter, that they have azoospermia, which means that there is no sperm in the ejaculate. Obviously, the presence of azoospermia makes natural conception impossible, but it's a condition that can possibly be corrected. Most patients think azoospermia means "no sperm, no hope," but patients with no sperm in their ejaculate may have sperm in a testicle that can be aspirated.

There are two types of azoospermia. The first is caused by an obstruction, and the second, which we saw in Dave's case, is nonobstructive azoospermia. In obstructive azoospermia, sperm may be produced in normal amounts, but because there is a blockage, no sperm end up in the ejaculate. In the latter, sperm production is insufficient within the testicle to get sperm into the ejaculate.

Nonobstructive azoospermia can be caused by a variety of factors. Some are genetic (for example, Klinefelter's Syndrome), and some are developmental, as when the testicles do not form properly, either in the fetus or at puberty. Another possible cause is toxic exposure—from chemotherapy, for example—after which, with time, some sperm production might resume. There may also be a lack of hormonal stimulation of the testicles from the pituitary, which is potentially correctable with medications.

As Dave discovered, just because there is no sperm present in the ejaculate does not mean that no sperm are being produced. Rather, it means that the number of sperm being produced in the testicle is inadequate to get sperm into the ejaculate. In fact, for those with nonobstructive azoospermia, overall, there is a 60 percent chance of finding adequate numbers of sperm for a successful IVF cycle.

The surgical technique that offers the best opportunity for finding sperm under these circumstances is called *testicular microdissection*. It is done in conjunction with ovarian stimulation of the female partner. This procedure, in which the testicles' tubules are carefully dissected under an operating microscope, is typically done in the operating room under a general anesthetic. It may be lengthy and tedious for the patient, but often it is the only way to assist with nonobstructive azoospermia. Because there is still a chance of failure even with this technique, the patient should decide in advance whether to have donor sperm available in a backup role. Typically, it takes 5 to 7 days for a patient to recover from this procedure, and he will be advised to take it easy for 2 weeks.

Obstructive azoospermia can either be congenital, caused by incomplete or incorrect development of the proper anatomic structures, or acquired, due to scarring from trauma or infection, or due to a vasectomy. There are two approaches to dealing with this: surgical correction of the blockage, or surgical retrieval of the sperm for use during IVF.

The most common surgically correctable blockage is one caused by a prior vasectomy that the patient wishes to reverse. This is known as a *vasovasostomy*, in which the ends of the vas deferens are surgically reattached. This is typically done in the operating room and is best accomplished with the aid of an operating microscope.

This is very delicate surgery—as any male might suspect—and is best performed by urologist with extensive experience with the procedure. Success rates of the procedure depend on the technical expertise of the surgeon, the time that has passed since the vasectomy was performed, the amount of scarring present from the vasectomy, and the presence of antisperm antibodies resulting from the vasectomy.

At times, when attempting to reconstruct the vas deferens, a *vaso-epididymostomy* will be required. In this procedure, the end of the vas deferens is connected to a tubule within the epididymis. This is necessary if there is inadequate flow of sperm in the proximal end of the vas deferens after the vasectomy.

The other option for those with obstructive azoospermia is a surgical sperm retrieval associated with IVF. Sperm retrieval is typically straightforward in these circumstances and can usually be accomplished under a local anesthetic by extracting fluid or tissue from either the epididymis or the testicle using a small hypodermic needle. Many viable sperm are typically obtained in this procedure, but because they are immature, they cannot fertilize a human ovum on their own, so they are used for intracytoplasmic sperm injection (ICSI) in association with IVF. This is the preferred treatment for men who've had a vasectomy in the distant past, those who have had a failed vasovasostomy, those with uncorrectable obstruction, or those whose female partner has concomitant infertility issues.

Men faced with infertility have to overcome emotional and physical challenges, but the fact is that they have a much better chance of fathering a child today than ever before. So, if you think your fertility may be in doubt, don't give up. There is a very good possibility that your challenges can be overcome. With modern medical knowledge, technology, and advanced surgical techniques, we are able to help the vast majority of our infertile male patients succeed in having children.

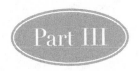

Part III

The Most
Common Solutions
and Preventions

CHAPTER TEN

The Donor
Sperm Option

SARA WAS A 38-year-old attorney in a prominent law firm when she became our patient. Sara had breezed through her undergraduate curriculum and then law school. She was made full partner in her firm at the age of 34, becoming the youngest female to ever attain that prestigious position.

Professionally, she was successful and accomplished. Personally, she was frustrated and concerned. She'd had several serious relationships but none was exactly right. She was career driven and always thought the opportunity would come along one day to have a family.

Then, Sara reached the age of 38 and realized her time for starting a family was running out. She decided that she would rather raise a child as a single parent than marry someone she did not love just to have a child. For these reasons, Sara was an ideal candidate for the sperm donor option.

Sara came to our clinic to ask about the donor sperm option, but she knew little about the treatment involved or how the process worked. We explained to her that we would do a basic fertility evaluation, which meant we would look at:

○ The quality of her eggs

○ Whether she was releasing an egg or ovulating monthly

○ The health of her uterus and fallopian tubes and their ability to carry out the necessary functions to conceive

This initial round of basic tests normally occurs within a month's time. During that period, we advised Sara to contact several of the top sperm banks in the country. Sperm banks have been operating in the United States since the early 1970s, and there are many reputable companies from which to choose.

Each year, thousands of people choose this option to overcome infertility or the lack of a suitable male partner. In this chapter, I will explain, as we did for Sara:

○ The recruitment and screening process for sperm donors

○ Reasons to use a sperm donor

○ The process for selecting donors with characteristics you are seeking

○ The evaluation of the woman for chances of pregnancy

○ Requirements to ensure your safety

○ Issues of disclosure with donor sperm

○ When the insemination isn't enough

○ Success rates using donor sperm

○ The risks involved

The Donors

Sperm donors are recruited in major metropolitan areas throughout the United States. Sperm donors come from all walks of life. They have varied ethnic backgrounds and education levels, and they have many different reasons for wanting to be a sperm donor. Many sperm donors want to donate for the compensation; others are more altruistic in their desire to help a woman realize her desire for pregnancy. Regardless of their reasons, the screening process remains the same—and it is quite rigorous.

Sperm donors are subjected to an extensive battery of tests and evaluation to ensure that they will be an excellent sperm source as well as a safe donor. Donors to sperm banks, or cryobanks, as they are also called, are usually required to be less than 40 years of age. They must undergo a general medical history screening and a physical examination to ensure that they have no underlying medical conditions. Mental health evaluations are also required. Sperm banks also check to see that donors lead a low-risk lifestyle that would not pre-dispose them to infectious diseases.

The donor's sperm are also tested through a semen analysis. The male must have excellent sperm parameters to be considered as a donor by a reputable sperm bank. Each donor is tested for genetic disorders such as cystic fibrosis, spinal muscular atrophy, thalassemia, and others that he may be at risk for based on his ancestry. Further, donors are given a chromosomal karyotype to evaluate their 23 chromosomes—this helps to ensure that they pass on normal chromosomes to a baby. They are tested for all known transmittable infectious diseases such as HIV, hepatitis B and C, syphilis, HTLV-I and II, gonorrhea, chlamydia, West Nile virus, and trypanosoma. Each year, the list of tested diseases is expanded to ensure the safety of the sperm recipient. All of these tests and examinations are done prior to any sperm being harvested from the donor.

Once donors pass this initial battery of testing, they are allowed to donate sperm. This is a serious commitment, because most sperm banks require them to donate two or three times per week over a 3- to 6-month period. In addition, they must be abstinent for 2 to 5 days before each collection.

Each sperm sample collected is quarantined for 6 months. At the end of each sperm collection, the donors are tested again for all of the transmittable infectious diseases to make sure they remain negative. This decreases the risk of transmitting these diseases to the recipient. There is a very low risk of contracting any of these diseases due to the stringent screening mandated by the US Food and Drug Administration.

After the donor's semen is collected, the sperm is isolated and frozen in small batches. If the sperm counts are very high, one semen collection can yield many vials of sperm to be used. Most vials of sperm have about 10 million to 20 million sperm in total—more than enough to result in a pregnancy. The sperm are frozen quickly with chemical protectants and stored in liquid nitro-gen at -196°C. Once frozen and stored, it can be stored for years without being compromised. Frozen sperm has been used after 20 years in storage and still resulted in a pregnancy. The sperm must remain frozen until use and must be transported from the cryobank in liquid nitrogen. Clinics often will keep the sperm frozen in a tank until a patient is ready to use it.

Most infertility clinics can store more than one specimen in liquid nitrogen tanks. Smaller clinics or general obstetrics-gynecology offices may not have such capability. Some may have to have their donor sperm sent overnight for use the following day. Be sure to check with your clinic to determine their policy regarding sperm shipping and storage and whether they maintain extra samples.

Is This the Option for You?

Why use a sperm donor? The list of women and couples who are candidates to use sperm donors continues to grow. Currently, these are the primary reasons that a woman or couple may use a donor:

○ Lack of a male partner—either single women or same-sex female couples

○ A male partner whose sperm are too poor in quality or low in number to conceive

○ A male partner who has an ejaculatory dysfunction that cannot be repaired

○ A male partner who has a sexually transmitted infection with a high risk of transmission to the female partner, such as HIV or hepatitis C

○ A severe blood type incompatibility between partners that would be harmful to a baby

○ A male partner who has an inheritable genetic disease that cannot be screened in any other way

○ A failed pregnancy or lack of embryo growth with the partner's sperm

Selecting a Donor

Sara selected an anonymous sperm donor from thousands of candidates. Her choice was made based on the characteristics and physical features she was looking for in a partner. Because she was not in a relationship, she used the image of her "perfect" partner—tall, blonde hair, dark eyes, with a professional background. It is not unusual for single women to seek sperm donors with traits reflecting their ideal mate—whether they be highly intellectual, Hollywood handsome, athletic, or well-rounded.

Some women have unique tastes, such as rock star Melissa Etheridge, who went for musical ability in her sperm donor, choosing another classic rock star, her friend David Crosby of Crosby, Stills and Nash. Lesbian mothers often try to match the characteristics of the sperm donor to their female partner in an effort to have a child similar to both parents. Heterosexual women often try to match the donor to their male partner in physical characteristics.

Out of thousands of sperm donors, how do you choose the best donor match for you? First and foremost, you should create of list of what you want in the donor. What are the most important characteristics of the donor—physical appearance? Personality? Athleticism? Intellect? Musical ability? Writing talent? Artistic ability?

Once you outline your goals, the search becomes easier. Most large sperm banks now have online search engines that aid you in narrowing down the list. You can enter your preferences for any physical characteristic, ethnic background, educational background into the search. You will receive a list of donors who meet your criteria, and then you can start the selection process. Some information is available for each donor, and you can often purchase photos, voice clips, personality inventories, and other aspects of their evaluation. This may give you a better insight into the donor to help decide who is right for you. Sara used the search engine and found six potential matches. She then viewed photos and selected the right donor for her.

Many sperm banks also offer a matching service to help you narrow the field even further. Couples who choose to use donor sperm and want a match to their male or female partner can submit a photo of the partner to the bank and ask them to find the person who most resembles them. The banks see the donors live and in person and can help match you up without searching through hundreds of donors to find the right fit. This is a great service for many couples.

Some couples also consider the option of selecting characteristics that they want. For example, our patient Joelle's husband, Michael, has always felt that he was too short at 5 feet 5 inches tall. Although he was a successful businessman, he felt that his life has been limited by his height. Unfortunately, he was found to have testicular failure, an irreversible condition that meant he didn't produce any sperm. They opted for donor sperm, and Michael wanted a tall donor so that his child might be taller than him. They chose a donor who was 6 feet tall.

This sort of "upgrade" often is frowned upon as unethical by some in the business because the medical goal of donor sperm programs is to help infertile couples have a child, not to create ideal children.

There are a few other medical and social considerations to decide upon when selecting the donor. How much sperm does the donor have in the bank? If the donor only has one or two vials available, bear in mind that it may take more than that to get pregnant. Also, are you considering more than one child? Do you want them to be genetically related from the same donor? It may be a good idea to purchase a larger number of sperm from a single donor and store some of it rather than using a donor with a limited supply—especially if you wish to have several children who are genetically similar.

You will also have to choose what type of sperm to use. The sperm banks process sperm in various ways to yield sperm that is prepared for intracervical insemination (ICI), intrauterine insemination (IUI), or in vitro fertilization (IVF). The amount of processing performed by the bank determines the cost per vial. For example, a specimen prepared for ICI is manipulated relatively little and therefore costs less. Sperm ready for IUI costs more because they have processed the specimen much more. Consult with your physician to determine which preparation is the best for you. If money is a concern, we recommend requesting the least expensive option that will suit your needs.

Anonymous and Open Donors

A relatively new dimension of sperm donation is the use of anonymous or open donors. An anonymous donor, as the name implies, remains anonymous and cannot be traced to the origin of the sperm. You may not contact the donor and, in return, he may never contact you.

With open donation, the donor has agreed to allow any children resulting to contact him either upon medical need or when the child reaches age 18. For some, this option is particularly appealing so that the child could, if desired, find their genetic parent. The donor still may not find the recipient in these cases. Because the donor sperm bank must keep in contact with the sperm donor for at least 18 years, the fee for the sperm is higher. Each sperm bank sets their own fees, and you should consult the bank of your choice to determine their rates.

Cytomegalovirus

Cytomegalovirus (CMV) is a very common and easily spread virus that is present in 80 percent of the population. Unfortunately, if a woman contracts CMV during pregnancy, it can be catastrophic, causing miscarriage, or blindness, deafness, mental retardation, and other birth defects. Checking a woman for their CMV status is relatively easy with a blood test. Because white blood cells are a method of transmission, women who are CMV negative should only receive sperm from a donor who is also CMV negative to avoid transmission during pregnancy.

If a woman is CMV positive, she may receive sperm from a donor who is either CMV positive or negative. The CMV status of the donor is often shown on the sperm bank's website or it is available as part of the donor's information.

The Friend Option

Sperm banks are just one way to obtain donated sperm. What if you have a male friend who is not your sexual partner but is willing to donate and assist with conception? This option is perfectly viable, but your friend must pass the same requirements that an anonymous donor is required to pass. This includes the sperm quarantine for 6 months. For some women, the prospect of knowing the donor is very important and worth the 6-month wait. For others, the 6-month quarantine period is just another unwanted hurdle in their attempts to get pregnant. Most sperm banks can assist you with the process of using a friend as your donor.

Making Sure You Can Carry
a Healthy Baby

Before you invest time, money, and emotions into a sperm donor, you should make certain that you can carry and give birth to a healthy baby. We told Sara, as we tell all of our clients, that she needed to ensure that she was healthy and fertile, too.

We recommended evaluation of Sara's fallopian tubes, uterus, and ovaries—the other key ingredients in creating a successful pregnancy. Sara underwent an x-ray of her uterus and tubes. This is the HSG (*hysterosalpingogram*) procedure. She was taken to the radiology department, where a small catheter was inserted through the cervix. We injected a small amount of fluid that shows up as a contrasting outline on the x-ray. When the fluid filled her uterus, Sara could look on the screen and see a triangular shape outlining her uterus. This confirmed that her uterus was normal. Seconds later, the fluid flowed out of the uterus into both fallopian tubes and then seemed to disappear into her peritoneal cavity, indicating that both tubes were open. Yet another good sign.

An ultrasound also was performed to evaluate Sara's ovaries and her uterus to confirm that Sara did not have any fibroids or other structural problems that might limit her chances of conception. Since Sara was 38, we did blood tests to confirm that the quality of her eggs was still good enough for a successful pregnancy. We also noted that her body was making enough progesterone hormones after ovulation to prepare the uterus for a baby.

The final step in Sara's examination was to make certain that she was free of any transmittable diseases before receiving donor sperm. The US Food and Drug Administration requires that tissue being transferred from one person to another must be screened for diseases. Besides the tissue, the person receiving it should be evaluated as well. Sara underwent testing for HIV, hepatitis B and C, syphilis, gonorrhea, and chlamydia. She was negative.

Once Sara's medical testing was complete, we determined that there were no obvious obstacles to her conceiving with the help of a sperm donor. She was on her way to starting her family. We'd taken care of the physical aspects of Sara's quest, but we also recommended that she speak with a psychologist to prepare herself for the mental and emotional aspects of this option.

The decision to use donor sperm is not one that should be taken lightly. Because it is a very important decision that will change your life, the American Society for Reproductive Medicine recommends consultation with a psychology professional trained in infertility. Besides helping to sort out the criteria that you have to select a donor, they often review the important issues of disclosure.

Who do you tell that you used donor sperm? Friends? Family? No one? The child? How do you tell them and when? There are ramifications to each decision, and the psychologist can help you sort them out and understand exactly what to expect. Keep in mind that there is no one right answer—only the answer that best serves your unique situation.

The Process for Using Donor Sperm

Once Sara selected her donor, his sperm was shipped frozen from the cryobank to our clinic. There it was held in liquid nitrogen until the day it was needed— the day of Sara's ovulation. At this point, it had been just 6 weeks since Sara's first visit to our clinic. Now, she was ready to begin her cycle of treatment, which could lead to conception within the month!

Sara became excited at that prospect and began calculating potential due dates for the birth of her baby. Once her period commenced she was instructed to report to the clinic on cycle day 12. Ultrasound and LH testing were initiated to track the development of her follicle. When her follicle achieved a diameter of approximately 20 millimeters, Sara noticed a color change in her home urine ovulation predictor test, revealing an LH surge. This indicated that she was going to ovulate the following day. She called the clinic and scheduled her day of insemination.

Sara arrived at the clinic on the designated morning. The frozen sperm she had selected was thawed, washed, and prepared in a small tube to be injected into her uterus. After inserting a speculum (as is done to perform a Pap smear), we threaded a small catheter through the cervix. We then injected into the uterus a small volume of fluid containing the washed, motile sperm.

Sara felt nothing except the speculum being removed. She was surprised to learn that the insemination process was over. She remained on the table for 5 minutes and then was able to go about her usual day. And so, the waiting began.

But Sara didn't have to wait long. Just 16 days later she realized her period was 2 days late. No cramps were good news in this case. Instead, Sara felt "strange," with some bloating and breast tenderness. A urine pregnancy test showed that she was pregnant!

When she called us to share the news, we told her to come in for a blood test the next day. We measured her hCG hormone, which showed a high level, suggesting that Sara was on her way to motherhood. Since her first pregnancy test, Sara enjoyed every minute of her pregnancy. The hallmarks of her journey included the first ultrasound with a heartbeat, the baby's kicking, the slow growth of her stomach, and finally the long-awaited birth. She delivered a very healthy baby girl, Sophia, who weighed 6 pounds, 10 ounces. Since her delivery, Sara's life has continued to change—for the better, in her opinion. Being a single mother, she has taken on a less hectic schedule at work and works 4 days per week instead of the previous 6 days per week. She has enjoyed her new little girl and all that she dreamed of having in her family. They have traveled to visit family and friends, and she enjoys showing off wonderful baby. She still visits me in the office regularly so I can watch Sophia grow as well.

We have come a long way in the use of donated sperm. Using frozen sperm for intrauterine insemination now produces the same pregnancy outcome as fresh sperm. The same percentage of women get pregnant with either method.

Sara was fortunate that she became pregnant during her first attempt. This is not always the case. The usual pregnancy rates for women less than 35 years of age, who use solely donor-sperm insemination without medications, is approximately 20 to 25 percent per month. With medications such as Clomid, the rate increases to 30 to 35 percent per attempt. Some women do not get pregnant even with these methods. When this happens, the options are either to select a different donor or to move forward with more aggressive therapy such as injectable medications or IVF. Depending on the age of the woman at the time she starts IVF, the pregnancy rates can be as high as 70 percent.

Using frozen sperm is especially appealing for women like Sara because of the decreased risk of HIV and other diseases that could be transmitted through fresh donor semen available in the 1970s. This practice has been abandoned with the advent of frozen sperm. With mandatory quarantining and screening for frozen sperm, there have been no recorded cases of women being infected with the HIV virus through donor sperm. Other risks, including transmission of other diseases, uterine cramping, and emotional aspects of the process, are minimal.

The donor sperm option has also proven to be a blessing for women in same-sex relationships. Our patients Julia and Niki had been together 4 years before deciding to start a family. Julia, 35, wanted to carry the child, "to experience the miracle of birth." Their first step was to pick a sperm donor, a process which they found to be "hilarious all in itself."

"We laughed hysterically at the question of how to hand-pick the 23 chromosomes for your child," Julia said. "At times, it felt more like we were picking out a new car and all of the accessories we ever wanted. But instead of four-wheel drive and a stereo, we were picking out our future child's hair color, eye color, detached or attached earlobes, thin or thick eyebrows, and of course whether we wanted the nostrils wide or narrow."

Once they selected a donor, Julia and Niki learned about the processes of buying, storing, shipping, washing, and adjusting the temperature of sperm "so that it is happy and productive," Julia said.

Next, they prepared for the first intrauterine insemination (IUI) with the help of one of our team, whom this good-natured couple dubbed "The Baby Planner."

"Thank goodness we had a baby planner, as the task of coordinating ovulation and the exact date of insemination required a lot of preparation and skill," Julia said. "We compared this stage to getting on a roller coaster and strapping yourself in."

The ups and downs included a failed first pregnancy test. Julia was then given Clomid to enhance development of the egg prior to a second insemination. Julia had hormone-induced mood swings while on this fertility drug. Again, she displayed good humor even when enduring this. "I called my evil twin 'CloMad,'" she said.

Julia had another negative pregnancy test, so we decided to pursue a more aggressive treatment and a "new adventure." We did a third IUI and this time administered fertility medications by injection. Niki took on the job of giving Julia one shot of the drug each day for 2 weeks.

"Niki quickly fine-tuned her shot-giving medical skills (even though she majored in psychology in college), and I learned to walk around twice day with a bag of frozen peas on my bottom," Julia said.

She notes that in the end, so to speak, the pain of the injections helped prep her for the pain of childbirth. "After 2 weeks of shots, we strapped ourselves back into the roller coaster, only to be disappointed," she said. "Again, we were not pregnant."

Three more failed attempts occurred. Niki and Julia met with our team and it was decided to give them a 6-month break before trying a new strategy. After six failed attempts, we concluded that the best approach was to go with in vitro fertilization.

"Just hearing the word 'infertility' was extremely difficult for me," Julia said. "But I felt I should try everything possible to become pregnant."

After a 6-month respite, Niki and Julia resumed the fertility shots and frozen peas routine; this time with two shots a day for 10 days.

"By this point I was pretty tough and didn't seem to mind the pain because I was so driven and had such high hopes of becoming pregnant," she said.

Our staff conducted an egg retrieval with Julia, and ultimately we transferred two embryos and froze another. After 2 days of bed rest and 2 weeks of waiting to take another pregnancy test, this couple finally received some good news. Julia was pregnant.

Their son Jaxson was born in the spring of 2009. Over his crib hangs the message, "Every child is a story yet to be told."

"Now that we have our son, the exhausting and emotional process of IUI and IVF is a faint memory," Julia said. "As we look at his big blue eyes, hear his laughter, and watch him discover the world, we know that it was all worth every second of the roller-coaster ride. It was the greatest challenge and the longest journey but we are so blessed that Jax's own story is one that is 'yet to be told.'"

Key Questions to Ask about the Donor Sperm Option

Here is a starter list of recommended questions for patients considering the sperm donor option to ask their doctors, clinic staff, and sperm banks.

○ Does the clinic have its own sperm bank?

○ If not, which sperm banks does the practice or clinic use?

○ Does the clinic provide a list of recommended sperm banks?

○ Does the clinic or sperm bank follow the donor sperm guidelines of American Society for Reproductive Medicine?

○ Does the sperm bank recommended follow all FDA guidelines?

○ Does the clinic have a storage tank available for frozen sperm?

○ Will the clinic reserve and store additional samples of the patient's donor for future cycles?

○ How much does it cost to store the sperm?

○ What testing do they recommend for donor sperm use?

○ What are my individual chances of success based on my testing?

CHAPTER ELEVEN

The Egg
Donor Option

THE RECIPIENT: MELANIE, 39, had been married to Jason for 15 years. They'd been trying to start a family for at least 10 years when she came to our clinic as a patient. Melanie had been having hot flashes, which had begun to increase in intensity.

During our evaluation, Melanie was found to be in premature menopause and there was no discernible way to stop it. Fortunately, we also found that Melanie's uterus was normal. Jason's evaluation was normal, too.

Melanie and Jason were eager to have children. We presented them with a variety of options, including egg donation and adoption. Melanie wanted to experience pregnancy and birth. Therefore, they chose to look for an egg donor. After much consideration, this couple opted to seek a donor through our clinic, which, like many, maintains a list of possible egg donors in our area.

Five months later, they were matched to the donor, whom they accepted based on the information in her profile. With our help, the two women then coordinated their menstrual cycles. The donor began the ovarian stimulation process and egg retrieval followed by fertilization in our laboratory with Jason's sperm. The embryos were then transferred to Melanie's uterus.

I am pleased to report that Melanie and Jason successfully conceived twins, a boy and a girl, delivered at 36 weeks. They are doing well and enjoying their long-awaited family, thanks to the egg donor option.

The donor: When Kim saw the unusual advertisement in her hometown newspaper, it struck an emotional chord. The ad was seeking women willing to donate their eggs to women unable to have children of their own. Kim had never heard of infertile women receiving donated eggs. She learned that medical science had only perfected methods for collecting donor eggs in the last few decades, but using donated eggs was becoming increasingly common, especially for women over the age of 40 who wanted to have children.

The more Kim thought about being an egg donor, the more it appealed to her, because of her loving relationship with her Aunt Katie, who had tried for many years but had been unable to have children of her own. "Her grief has always had an impact on me, for she would have been an excellent mother," Kim said.

Kim saw egg donation as an opportunity not only to help another woman become a mother but to also honor the memory of her beloved aunt, who had given so much to her as a child. Then, of course, she had to face the reality that being an egg donor is a time-consuming and sometimes scary process. There were needles involved, which did not thrill her.

Still, Kim found that donating eggs was far more rewarding than she had imagined. "I received an incredible letter from the egg recipient," she said. "I cried all the way home knowing of the joyous impact I was making on another woman's life."

A year later, Kim became an egg donor for the second time, and there was no letdown. "My experience was even better because I knew that I was being inspired from within to help someone who would hopefully know the joy of motherhood," she said.

Many men and women who feared they would never have children also feel inspired by the experience. They are grateful that a donor's eggs made it possible for them to be parents.

In this chapter, we will provide insights into and information about infertility treatments using donated eggs. This procedure, while relatively new, has become increasingly popular and very successful.

Success rates from donated eggs vary from clinic to clinic. In 2007, our clinic completed 217 egg donor transfer cycles and 177 resulted in pregnancies, for a success rate of 81.6 percent. Donor eggs (*oocytes*) have become a very viable option for women who may have no other chance to become pregnant. This treatment can lead to successful pregnancies for women with any of the following fertility challenges:

○ Premature ovarian failure or early menopause

○ Eggs of poor quality (judged by decreased egg counts or by a poor IVF cycle)

○ Older reproductive age group (but still under age 50)

○ Chromosomal translocations or genetic diseases that they wish to avoid passing on to their offspring

The decision to use an egg donor can be very easy for some, such as those faced with premature ovarian failure, and very difficult for others, such as those who have poor quality eggs. Most women would prefer to use their own eggs. After exhausting all options with their own eggs through either IVF, alternative therapies like acupuncture, or considerable time trying, some decide to use donor eggs as their only hope for having children. With the egg donor option, the egg is extracted from the donor, then fertilized in vitro and transferred to the recipient.

We find that once a woman or a couple accepts donor eggs as an option, they embrace the idea and move forward knowing that they have tried everything in their power to conceive on their own.

Obtaining donor eggs is much more difficult than using donor sperm. Currently, eggs must be retrieved fresh and used fresh, whereas donor sperm can be frozen for decades and obtained from sperm banks. Until recently, egg freezing has not been successful and therefore was not a viable option. In coming years, we expect this to change with the increasing success of a rapid egg-freezing method known as egg *vitrification* (see Chapter 13). With this method, donor egg banks will likely begin to emerge and greatly simplify the process, just as sperm banks have done for sperm donation.

Because of the invasive nature of egg donation, finding a donor may be a difficult process. Being an egg donor is time-consuming, invasive, and requires many office visits and injections as well as blood draws. The donor must be totally committed to the process because of all that is required of her.

Egg donation often takes time away from the donor's everyday life or work. Donors are compensated for their time, which may represent a motivation for some. In our program, first-time donors are compensated $5,000 and repeat donors receive $5,500. By contrast, the average sperm donor receives approximately $50 to $100 per sperm collection for a much less invasive donation.

How can you adequately pay someone for giving you their life-giving eggs? The answer is that you cannot. Their compensation is solely for their time and effort expended during the cycle. Recipients cannot buy eggs—they can only compensate the donors for their time. According to the American Society for Reproductive Medicine (ASRM), "monetary compensation of the donor should reflect the time, inconvenience, and physical and emotional demands and risks associated with oocyte donation and should be at a level that minimizes the possibility of undue inducement of donors and the suggestion that payment is for the oocytes themselves."

Ads in an early 1990s newspaper offered $50,000 for the perfect donor—clearly an excessive amount. This excess is strongly frowned upon by most, if not all, legitimate infertility centers and by the ASRM. Egg donors typically spend an average of 40 to 50 hours total in the standard procedures. The time spent includes driving to and from the clinic and having various medical evaluations, injections, and procedures, and may require the donor to miss work.

With all this investment by the donor, how do you find someone willing to step up to help you? There are three typical egg donor sources: a friend or family member, an anonymous donor recruited through a donor agency, or an anonymous donor recruited by your fertility clinic.

Each option has particular advantages and disadvantages and should be weighed carefully before selecting a donor.

Finding a Donor among Friends or Family

The friends and family option has many excellent benefits. The egg donor is well known to you and may even be genetically linked. The process tends to be quicker and less expensive because you don't usually have to pay them.

The downside of a friend or family member as a donor is that relationship issues often surface during or after pregnancy. To save you both grief, you and your family or friend egg donor should have heart-to-heart discussions early on about what sort of relationship they'll want with you and the child after birth. For example, if your sister is your egg donor, will she be satisfied to merely serve as the child's aunt, or will she feel more like a mother to the child? If she feels more motherly, this could lead to conflicts with you as you raise the child.

This conversation may be difficult, but it is necessary to avoid conflicts and misunderstandings later. You should work through what you want and what they want and what both sides expect. One pair of sisters, Paula and Amanda, whom we worked with a few years ago, had this discussion and found that they wanted the same thing: a child for the recipient and a niece for the donor. It worked out beautifully.

A more recent pair of sisters, Cassie and Samantha, realized that the prospective egg donor, Cassie, just wasn't comfortable knowing that the potential recipient, Samantha, would have a child that would be Cassie's own flesh and blood. Samantha saw that there could be conflicts with her sister, so she opted for an anonymous donor.

Egg Donor Agencies

The second option for a donor is to use one of the many donor agencies around the country. An egg donor agency recruits and retains donors all over the United States. Various agencies focus on recruiting different types of donors. For example, an agency in New York specifically recruits only donors of Asian descent, while another agency in California seeks intellectually gifted donors with high IQ scores. You have a much larger pool to draw from by using an agency to find a donor, and choice is often touted as one of the best benefits of this option. Most agencies are reputable and recruit high-quality donors. You should check them out by asking for references and talking to people who have used them.

Another benefit of using an agency is that the process is often faster than with other options. The downside is cost; the agencies charge a fee for finding the donor. Some donors may command a higher fee based on their characteristics and occupation. There also may be travel fees to pay depending on your egg donor's location and the agency's distance from your clinic. Each agency has its own fee scale. We advise you to carefully check out any agency you choose to deal with before you sign an agreement with them. Keep in mind that some fees, regardless of whether you use their donor, are non-refundable.

Clinic Donors

The final option is to use a donor recruited by your fertility clinic, usually from within the surrounding area. Donors are often college students, young professionals, or young mothers. There is usually less expense incurred using your clinic's donor program because donors' compensation is fixed, without travel or agency fees. At our clinic, we offer photos of the donor as a child but not as adults because we want to protect their identities and most of them live in our area. The goal is to offer donor listings similar to the big national donor agencies. We have an on-line database for recipients to choose their own donor and search for the characteristics they want.

If you decide to use a friend or family member or a donor provided by an agency, you select the donor and your clinic performs medical screening to ensure your safety and that of your donor. When our patients use a donor from our clinic's pool, they are matched to the donor based on the patient's requests and requirements. Most women or couples look for a physical match with their donor. Others require qualities like musical ability, intelligence, or athleticism.

Couples hoping to match specific ethnic groups can have a tougher time finding a donor. It could take up to a year to find a match.

Whatever the criteria, our program works hard to match the patient as closely as possible to her "perfect" donor. Once matched, the patient reviews the donor's profile and decides if she is right. If the match is made, the process begins and, if not, we keep looking for an acceptable donor.

Many patients looking for egg donors find themselves pondering the age-old question of nature or nurture. Will choosing an egg donor with musical ability necessarily help you to have a musical child? Does a donor's high intelligence guarantee that your child will ace organic chemistry in college? Or does family environment have more to do with a child developing certain talents and abilities?

We can't give you those answers. Science has struggled with the nature-nurture question for generations. If you believe nature, then you will seek a donor with the qualities that you want exemplified. If you feel the environment decides their fate, choose a good physical match and raise your child in the setting that suits you best.

In our egg donor program, all donors on our list must be screened and ready for donation as soon as you accept them. This saves the heartache that may occur if the "perfect" woman doesn't pass her screening and is then ineligible to be your donor.

Screening the Donor

The screening for our program is very rigorous, and on average, we accept only one out of ten donors we screen. For a friend or family member, the acceptance criteria and allowable age range are less restricted. We look for friends and family donors who are between 19 and 40 years old, but preferably less than 35 years old. For an anonymous donor, the recommended range is between 19 and 33 years old.

The screening for anonymous donors at most infertility clinics requires the following:

○ A medical history and physical exam with a physician to assess their general well-being

○ Testing for infectious diseases including HIV, hepatitis B and C, syphilis, gonorrhea, chlamydia, cytomegalovirus, West Nile virus, and trypanasoma, in accordance with the US Food and Drug Administration guidelines

○ Illicit drug screening

○ Chromosomal karyotype

○ Screening for inheritable diseases such as cystic fibrosis, thalassemia, and spinal muscular atrophy based on ethnic ancestry

○ Review of two generations of family health history by a genetic counselor and physician to evaluate for inheritable diseases

○ Evaluation of egg quality and quantity

○ Psychological assessment by personality inventory questionnaire and inter-view with a psychologist

Evaluation of the recipient woman or couple occurs while they are finding the right donor. We want to be sure that there is no condition other than poor egg quality affecting their fertility. The evaluation for the recipient includes a thorough assessment of the uterus—a key factor in the donor egg process. The uterus is evaluated by ultrasound for evidence of fibroids, polyps, or other structural abnormality. Blood flow to the uterus is reviewed by uterine artery Doppler—a very specialized ultrasound that determines how well blood is flowing.

An office *hysteroscopy* is performed to evaluate the inside of the uterine cavity and to determine whether there is any scarring or other abnormality present. The final test is a functional assessment of the uterus called a mock cycle—the woman uses estrogen to build the lining of the uterus, just as she will when the real cycle begins. This test ensures that the uterus will respond properly during the procedure.

The male partner will also put in his share of time at the clinic. It is critical to evaluate his sperm, or that of the sperm donor in the case of single women or lesbian couples. Both the male and female will also be tested for transmitta-ble infections such as HIV, hepatitis, and syphilis.

All parties involved will also be given psychological assessments, because egg donation and pregnancy are major life changes, in both wondrous and stressful ways. The psychological evaluation is performed by a counselor trained in infertility issues. The patients are given guidance for dealing with this process.

The Fertilization and Incubation Process

Once both the donor and the recipient have completed the screening, the process begins. In order to coordinate the women's cycles, birth control pills are often used by the donor and the recipient. Strange as it may seem, the Pill is crucial because it helps us align the menstrual cycles effectively. Once the process is underway, the donor receives injected medications to stimulate the ovaries. This is done under close monitoring at the clinic. Simultaneously, the recipient starts the estrogen again to build the uterine lining. After 9 to 14 days of stimulation, the donor undergoes her egg retrieval—an outpatient surgical procedure to "harvest" the eggs. Her eggs are then fertilized in the laboratory with sperm (either the recipient's partner's, or donor sperm), and the resulting embryos are grown in a culture for 3 or 5 days. This is an exciting time because the possibility of pregnancy is a mere few weeks away.

Once fertilization and incubation have been completed, one or two embryos are transferred to the recipient's uterus. The number of embryos transferred usually depends on the donor's age and success rate. Once transferred, the long, 9- to 14-day wait begins to determine whether a pregnancy will result. This waiting period can be the most grueling stage of all, so we recommend that you plan some activities to take your mind off what's going on in your body, if that is possible.

Often, there are extra embryos available after transfer to the uterus. These may be frozen for use later on, either if a pregnancy doesn't occur or if you would like more children. Freezing embryos gives you the chance to have genetically related children without repeating the entire process. Although there are frequently extra embryos to freeze, this is not always the case. Extra embryos are a bonus that we strive for with each donor cycle. If there are none, an egg donor is sometimes willing to donate again to a couple who have used her eggs, so that the children will be genetically related.

The Egg Donor's Risks

Most women who donate their eggs do so without any complications, and they return to their pre-donation health status within a few days. Still, as with any procedure, there are risks involved to the egg donor. Because the egg retrieval is a surgical procedure, there is a minimal amount of risk due to the surgery or anesthesia. The risks include bleeding or infection and may require other surgery to stop any bleeding that may occur.

Another risk of donating eggs is *ovarian hyperstimulation syndrome* (OHSS). This is a rare complication of ovarian stimulation, and there are methods to help prevent this from occurring. Often, it can be treated by bed rest and increased fluids.

Studies have shown no increased risk of cancer or long-term side effects associated with the fertility medications administered during the donor cycle. However, because these studies were performed for no more than six donor cycles, donors are limited to six donations, in accordance with ASRM recommendations.

Each woman is born with 6 to 7 million eggs. By the time each she reaches puberty, she has approximately 500,000 eggs. Thus, donating a small number to another woman does not decrease the donor's chance of conceiving a child in the future, nor will it make her reach menopause sooner. Each month, a woman's ovaries prepare 10 to 30 eggs for stimulation—if they are not stimulated, they will die. The eggs that are stimulated are those that would have been used that month regardless and, therefore, the donor is not losing any extra eggs.

The approximate cost of donor egg IVF in our program, including donor workup, medications, and an anonymous egg donor cycle is $29,000 to $33,000. The entire process, from evaluation to the actual transfer, can take from 2 to 9 months to complete.

One of our patients, Wendy, was very concerned about the time element because she feared she was getting too old to have children. She was very relieved at how quickly the process went once she decided to use an egg donor. Wendy has graciously offered to share her story with you, in her own words.

WENDY'S STORY

I didn't marry until I was 44, and while I had always wanted children, I'd come to believe that it wasn't possible because of my age. However, my husband and I did speak to my doctor about possible fertility treatments, and initially we were referred to a medical center that was not operated by Dr. Schoolcraft.

I was placed on Clomid [clomiphene citrate], but only after undergoing a laparoscopy and hysterosalpingogram to ensure there were no problems with my uterus or fallopian tubes. I recall being very excited the first time I started the medication, as I was convinced I would be pregnant almost straightaway. But in truth, I spent month after month taking my temperature daily to chart my cycle, taking my medication, and trying to determine when I was ovulating so my husband and I could have sex!

The sadness and disappointment I felt each month when my period arrived was all-consuming. Time after time, I allowed myself to feel excited, and I even took some pregnancy tests! But the outcome was always the same: I wasn't pregnant.

After more than a year, I decided I could no longer continue with the cycle of failure and disappointment. My doctor suggested that I had two options: I could seek further help through in vitro fertilization (IVF), or simply accept that at my age, I was not going to be a mother. IVF is very expensive, and at first we didn't think it was an option for us, but thanks to my father-in-law's generosity, we were able to pursue it.

I already understood that I might have to use a donor egg, and I had no problems with that, but we all agreed we did not want to use a surrogate. I met with Dr. Schoolcraft, and he agreed to treat me if I passed all the medical tests. The very next day I made an appointment to do the tests. I passed every single one.

Next, we had psychological counseling to prepare ourselves for using a donor, and we certainly had no qualms about that. I knew it was our only chance of getting pregnant, and at the end of the day, I would be carrying the baby, so as far as we were concerned, the baby would be ours.

That April we were advised we had been matched with a donor from the clinic's file. I started on medication and shots to coordinate our cycles. I was told this could take up to 6 months. In May, my donor and I were in synch, and the process of retrieving her eggs and fertilizing them with my husband's sperm began. We elected to use a procedure in which a single sperm is injected into the egg to fertilize it (intracytoplasmic sperm injection, or ICSI).

Two weeks later, I visited the hospital for a pregnancy test, having already done one at home that had been positive. When the nurse called me to give me the results of the hospital test, she said I must be having twins because my hormone levels were so high! She was correct. I had fraternal twin boys. Jamie and Oliver are now 4½ years old! So there is hope—many other women of my age have undertaken donor egg IVF and been successful in starting their families, too.

Chapter Twelve

In Vitro Fertilization

On his first day of kindergarten, with his mother, Kelly, and other parents in the classroom, Chad was called on by his new teacher.

"Tell us your name and something interesting about yourself," the teacher asked him.

"My name is Chad," the boy said, "and I was a frozen embryo."

Chad's stunned teacher immediately looked at his mother, who smiled calmly and whispered, "I'll explain later."

Chad's story is no longer unique. *Time* magazine reported in January of 2009 that more than 3.5 million "test tube babies" had so far been conceived through in vitro fertilization (IVF). IVF has been the answer to the prayers of millions of men and women who otherwise might not have been able to conceive. Yet it is a complex procedure, and only about one-fourth of all IVF attempts with fresh female eggs result in a healthy birth. The odds of success using IVF with frozen eggs are lower, around 17 percent, according to the *Time* report. Still, improved methods and procedures are being developed all the time in our clinic and others around the world.

Kelly's case is fairly typical. She was a track and cross-country runner in high school and then in college, where she earned a degree as a registered nurse specializing in psychology. In her early twenties, she married another outstanding athlete, and they made plans to start a family.

From the beginning, Kelly had concerns about her ability to have children. Her career as a runner and her lean body mass had affected her menstrual cycles, which were irregular when she was still competing. Kelly knew from her medical training that she had to increase her body fat in preparation for bearing children. She did that by cutting back on her running. Despite her efforts, she could not carry a baby full term.

"After my fifth miscarriage, I found my husband crying on the floor, and I lay down and cried with him," she said. "He told me that he felt helpless because he couldn't give me the baby we wanted so badly."

Frustrated and frightened, Kelly came to our clinic when she was still in her twenties. She was already in a demanding job as head nurse of a major psychiatric center in the Denver area. Kelly impressed us with her intelligence—and with her determination, when she declared: "I will never be okay until I can have children."

We could see that the stress was taking a toll on this young woman. Kelly, who had always prided herself on her self-discipline, had managed to acquire six speeding tickets in several months. She told me that she had also broken down in tears during a meeting with her supervisors "for no apparent reason."

Her battle with infertility had left Kelly feeling that her life was "spinning out of control," she said. We assured her that we would do our best to help her regain a sense of control as we worked to help her have a child.

Over several months, we did a complete workup with extensive tests and found that Kelly had a complex set of physical challenges, which we traced, in part, to an undiagnosed and untreated infection from her teen years. She'd had a blighted ovum, a condition in which a fertilized egg attaches itself to the uterine wall but the embryo does not develop. Then we discovered she'd had an ectopic pregnancy that resulted in a ruptured fallopian tube. Her doctors had to remove that tube and then close off the other one because they feared future infections in it.

"When you are only 26 years old and childless and your doctor says he has to tie off your only remaining tube, it's a devastating thing to hear," Kelly recalled.

We explained that given her complex set of medical challenges, her best hope for sustaining a pregnancy was in vitro fertilization, then a relatively new method for dealing with infertility. This process for fertilizing a woman's egg cells outside her womb had resulted in the first successful birth of "test tube babies" just 8 years earlier, in 1978. When Kelly underwent her in vitro fertilization, the success rate was only about 13 percent. Today, our clinic has a success rate of 60 percent for in vitro fertilization treatments.

We are happy to report that Kelly's son Chad, now in his late teens, was one of our early success stories. And Kelly became a repeat customer, too. A few years later, she underwent a second in vitro fertilization, which gave the world Dillon, also now a teenager.

I keep close tabs on all of my patients and former patients, but Kelly and her boys stay closer than most. Because of her personal experiences and her training as a psychological nurse, we asked Kelly to join our clinic's team. Today, she shares her story with our patients and guides them through their own fights for fertility as our patient advocate.

IVF is one of the most successful treatments for infertility, yet it's also one of the most expensive and sometimes controversial. It is literally a method for achieving fertilization outside the body.

In most cases, IVF is the best hope for women with endometriosis, immunological challenges, unexplained infertility, and blocked or irreparably damaged fallopian tubes. IVF is also sometimes prescribed for women whose male partners are infertile.

In Vitro Fertilization: The Basics

The birth of Louise Brown, the first "test tube baby," was big news in 1978. She was the first child to have been conceived by in vitro fertilization. Today, the procedure is one of many assisted reproductive techniques (ART) available for people who want to have children. Since Louise entered the world to great fanfare, thousands of babies have been conceived and born each year with the help of these same techniques. In fact, IVF babies account more than 1 percent of all babies born in the United States; in Denmark, more than 5 percent of all newborns are IVF babies.

In vitro is a Latin term that translates to "in the glass." The term refers to procedures done outside the body, in a laboratory or other artificial environment. In IVF, a man's sperm and a woman's eggs are combined in a laboratory dish. One or more fertilized eggs (embryos) may be transferred to the woman's uterus, where they may implant in the uterine lining and develop. Excess embryos may be frozen, or *cryopreserved*, for future use.

The basic steps in an IVF treatment cycle (see Figure 1) are

1. Ripening the eggs (*ovarian stimulation*)

2. Retrieving the eggs

3. Fertilizing the eggs

4. Growing the embryos

5. Transferring the embryos to the uterus

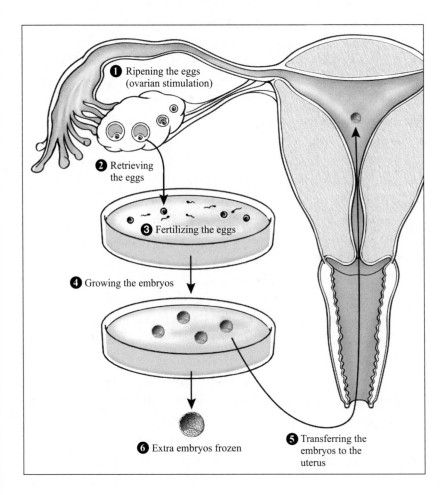

❶ Ripening the eggs (ovarian stimulation)

❷ Retrieving the eggs

❸ Fertilizing the eggs

❹ Growing the embryos

❺ Transferring the embryos to the uterus

❻ Extra embryos frozen

Figure 1: Process of in vitro fertilization

Step One: Ripening the Eggs (Ovarian Stimulation)

A woman's eggs develop inside fluid-filled sacs, called *follicles*, inside the ovaries. During a natural menstrual cycle, several follicles begin to enlarge, around the time when the woman is having her period.

However, over the course of the next few weeks, only one of these follicles develops to maturity; it then ruptures and releases its egg during the process of ovulation. The other follicles that had begun to develop then stop growing and dissolve. Therefore, only a small percentage of eggs present in the ovaries are ovulated during the woman's reproductive life span.

During IVF, our goal is for the patient to produce as many healthy, viable eggs as possible so we can retrieve them for fertilization. We can "rescue" follicles and eggs that would otherwise degenerate by giving shots of fertility drugs which contain FSH (*follicle-stimulating hormone*). This is the same hormone that the pituitary gland produces to cause one egg to develop. If we increase the woman's blood level of FSH, several follicles may grow at approximately the same rate, which allows us to collect more than one mature egg.

The first fertility drug that most women use is Lupron (leuprolide acetate). This drug causes the pituitary gland to release high amounts of FSH and LH (*luteinizing hormone*) for several days until its stores are depleted. Since continued use of Lupron prevents the pituitary gland from producing new supplies of FSH and LH, the amount of these hormones being released per day becomes very low after 7 to 10 days. We prescribe Lupron to ensure that blood levels of LH are low during the last few days of follicle growth, since we know that high levels of LH can lead to poor egg quality and stimulate progesterone production by the ovaries. A premature rise in progesterone may cause inappropriate maturation of the uterine lining and reduce the chance that the embryo will implant.

Some women will be placed on a Lupron "flare" medication schedule. This involves starting Lupron early in the menstrual cycle after suppressing pituitary and ovarian function for up to 1 month using birth control pills. The Lupron causes a sudden flare in the FSH and LH released by the pituitary gland, which initiates follicular growth.

On the third day after the Lupron starts, the woman begins shots of FSH or FSH and LH. (Brand names include Repronex, Follistim, and Gonal-F.) This stimulates the continued growth of the follicles as the pituitary's release of FSH begins to decline. Women over age 39 and those with high day-3 FSH blood levels are typically treated with a Lupron "flare" schedule in order to maximally stimulate the ovaries. Repronex (menotropins), Follistim (follitropin beta), or Gonal-F (follitropin alpha) is administered by injection.

Younger women or those with polycystic ovary syndrome (see Chapter 4) are usually treated with Lupron for approximately 10 days prior to beginning the shots of FSH. On this "long Lupron" schedule, the pituitary gland is no longer releasing large amounts of LH and FSH when Repronex, Follistim, or Gonal-F is started. The best treatment schedule is determined by the unique circumstances of the individual patient. The average number of follicles that develop is between 8 and 25, although some women will have more than 30 and others will develop less than 5.

Another class of drugs, called *gonadotropin-releasing hormone* (GnRH) *antagonists* (under the brand names Antagon and Cetrotide), may be used in some patients over a shorter time to prevent a spontaneous LH surge and ovulation without overly suppressing ovarian function.

With either the Lupron flare or the long Lupron schedule, the Repronex, Follistim, or Gonal-F shots are administered twice daily for 8 to 11 days, depending on how quickly the follicles mature. We can assess the ovarian response to these fertility drugs by measuring the follicle sizes with vaginal ultrasound and by following the increase in production of estradiol (estrogen) and progesterone by the cells inside the follicles. When the largest follicles reach approximately 18 millimeters in diameter, the woman takes a shot of hCG (*human chorionic gonadotropin*, which is sold under the brand names Profasi and Pregnyl). This hormone stimulates the final steps of maturation of the eggs. The egg collection occurs 35 hours after the hCG injection (see Figure 2).

Clomid (clomiphene citrate) is administered orally while the other medications listed are given by injection.

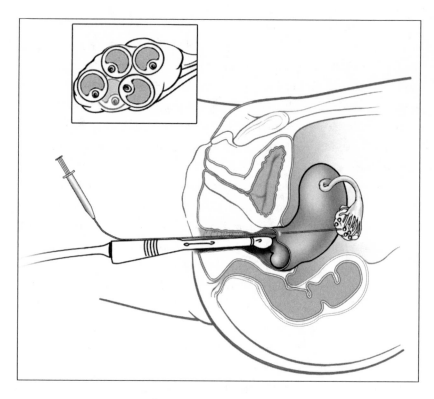

Figure 2: Oocyte retrieval

Step Two: Retrieving the Eggs

The Follicles

Using ultrasound examinations and blood testing, the physician can determine when the follicles are appropriate for egg retrieval. These tests can determine when the follicles have grown to the point that the egg inside is mature and ready for harvest (usually 8 to 12 days after the start of the treatment). When the follicles are ready, hCG or other medications are given. The hCG replaces the woman's natural LH surge and causes the final stage of egg maturation so the eggs can be fertilized. The eggs are retrieved before ovulation occurs, usually 34 to 36 hours after the hCG injection is given.

As many as 20 percent of IVF cycles may be cancelled prior to egg retrieval. This occurs for a variety of reasons, but usually it is due to an inadequate number of follicles developing. Cancellation rates due to low response to the ovulation drugs increase with age, especially after age 35. When cycles are cancelled due to a poor response, alternate drug strategies may be helpful to promote a better response in future attempts. Occasionally, a cycle may be cancelled to reduce the risk of *ovarian hyperstimulation syndrome* (OHSS).

Treatment with a GnRH antagonist reduces the possibility of premature LH surges from the pituitary gland, and thereby reduces the risk of premature ovulation. However, LH surges and ovulation occur prematurely in a small percentage of ART cycles despite the use of these drugs; if it does, the cycle is usually cancelled, since it is unknown when the LH surges began and when eggs will mature.

The Eggs

Egg retrieval is usually accomplished by *transvaginal ultrasound aspiration*, a minor surgical procedure that can be performed in the physician's office or an outpatient center under sedation by an anesthesiologist. A sterile vaginal ultrasound probe is used to guide a needle through the vaginal wall and into the follicle of the ovary (see Figure 2). Although it is long, the needle is not much wider than a needle used to draw blood from an arm vein.

Once the needle is inside the follicle, suction is created to pull the egg and the fluid through the needle and into a collection tube. When one follicle is drained, the needle is gently repositioned to collect fluid from each adjacent follicle. This is done for both ovaries. The follicular fluid is given to the embryologist, who examines it under a microscope to find the eggs. The entire procedure takes approximately 20 minutes. After an hour of observation in the recovery room, patients are allowed to return to their home or hotel.

Some women experience cramping on the day of the retrieval, but this sensation usually subsides by the next day. Women may also have feelings of fullness or pressure, which may last for several weeks following the procedure if the ovaries remain enlarged. In some circumstances, one or both ovaries may be inaccessible by transvaginal ultrasound. In rare circumstances, *laparoscopy* may then be used to retrieve the eggs using a small telescope inserted through the navel.

Step Three: Fertilizing the Eggs

The male partner provides the laboratory with a semen specimen to be used for fertilization of the eggs, unless donor or frozen sperm are being used. With normally functioning sperm, the eggs and several thousand sperm are placed together in a dish that contains a nutrient liquid. These dishes are kept in an incubator overnight and are examined under the microscope on the morning after the egg retrieval to determine which eggs have fertilized normally.

An alternative method of achieving egg fertilization is *intracytoplasmic sperm injection*, or ICSI. An extremely sharp glass needle is used to inject one sperm directly into the center (*cytoplasm*) of the egg under the guidance of a specially fitted microscope (see Figure 3). Candidates for ICSI include men with

○ severely compromised sperm parameters, including concentration, motility, or morphology, or antisperm antibodies

○ blockage or absence of the vas deferens, in which case sperm are surgically collected by epididymal aspiration or testicular biopsy for ICSI

○ low or failed fertilization on prior IVF attempts

○ unexplained infertility

The success rate with ICSI varies considerably among IVF programs and is highly dependent upon the skill of the embryologist performing the procedure.

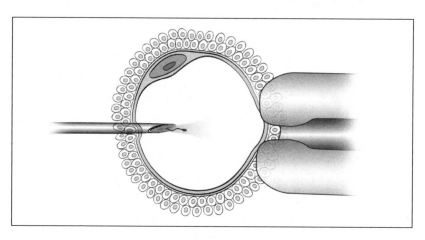

Figure 3: Intracytoplasmic sperm injection (ICSI)

In the United States, ICSI is performed in approximately 60 percent of ART cycles. Overall, pregnancy and delivery rates with ICSI are similar to the rates seen with traditional IVF. Genetic counseling is advisable before ICSI if inherited abnormalities are identified that may be passed to the child from the father.

The following day we examine the eggs by microscope to confirm fertilization. Approximately 40 percent to 70 percent of the mature eggs will fertilize after insemination or ICSI sperm injection. Lower rates may occur if the sperm or egg quality is poor. Occasionally, fertilization does not occur at all, even if sperm injection was used.

Handle with Care

One of the most important aspects of a successful IVF cycle is the handling of the eggs and embryos outside of the body. Among standard protocols is to use a sequence of culture media—the substance in the lab dish where we place the eggs and embryos—designed to physiologically resemble the environment in the female body, which changes throughout the development process. In other words, the eggs and embryos need different things at different times, and our sequential media matches those changes that occur in the female body.

Reproducing the human environment helps to minimize stress on the embryo, which is necessary for a positive outcome. Specialized environmental conditions are maintained in the IVF laboratory to eliminate contaminants and volatile substances in the air which may adversely affect embryos. A state-of-the-art IVF laboratory such as the one at our clinic is hermetically sealed and pressurized with a positive pressure system and advanced air filtration system designed to remove 99.9 percent of particulate matter.

Step Four: Growing the Embryos

After 2 days, the fertilized egg has divided to become a two- to four- cell embryo. By the third day, a normally developing embryo will contain approximately 6 to 10 cells (see Figure 4).

Although embryos may be transferred to the uterus at any time between 1 to 6 days after the egg retrieval, traditionally, the majority of embryo transfers are performed after 3 days of culture, when the embryos have 6 to 10 cells. The embryo first moves into the uterus at about 80 hours after ovulation. The

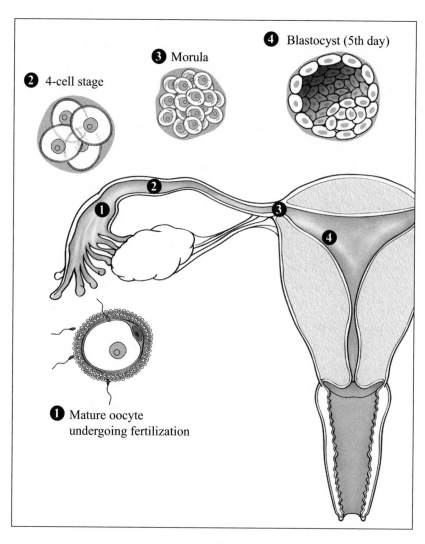

Figure 4: Stages of embryo development

implantation process begins about 3 days later, after the embryo has reached the blastocyst stage (usually around day 5 after fertilization) and hatching has occurred. Many embryos that appear to be healthy on day 3 fail to develop in the laboratory to blastocysts. Often programs transfer more embryos on day 3 than they would on day 5 to compensate for the fact that some day 3 embryos will stop developing before the blastocyst stage.

By the fifth day, a fluid cavity forms in the embryo, and the placenta and fetal tissues begin to separate. By choosing the optimal blastocysts for transfer on day 5, it's possible to select the embryos with the highest potential for implanting and making a baby. The day 5 embryos are more developed and have a better chance for maturing, so we have worked to develop ways to use them instead of day 3 embryos.

If successful development continues in the uterus, the embryo hatches from the surrounding "shell" or outer membrane, called the *zona pellucida*, and implants into the lining of the uterus approximately 6 to 10 days after the egg retrieval.

Assisted Hatching

In order for the advanced embryo to implant in the uterine wall and to continue development, it must break free of its zona pellucida or shell. Some embryos grown in the laboratory may have a harder shell than normal or may lack the energy needed to complete the hatching process. The embryologists can help these embryos achieve successful implantation through a technique called *assisted hatching*.

On the third day of laboratory growth and shortly prior to uterine transfer, a small hole is made in the shell of the embryo with a specially fitted microscope. Through this opening, the cells of the embryo can escape from the shell and implant at a somewhat earlier time of development, when the uterine lining may be more favorable.

Women who are most likely to benefit from assisted hatching are those

O Over 38 years of age

O With mild elevations in their day 3 FSH levels

O With repeated failures of ART cycles or

O With embryos that have abnormal-looking shells, as determined through close inspection by the embryologists

The skill of the embryologist is extremely important when hatching is performed. Our embryologists have performed this technique for many years and have found it to improve pregnancy and delivery rates for patients whose prognoses are otherwise poor.

Genetic Screening

Preimplantation genetic diagnosis (PGD) is performed at some centers to screen for inherited diseases. During this process (described in greater detail in Chapter 16), one or two cells are removed from the developing embryo and tested for specific genetic diseases, such as cystic fibrosis and Down syndrome. Embryos that do not show signs of disease are selected for transfer to the uterus. These procedures require specialized equipment and experience.

Some couples want to use this method to screen the embryos for disease even if they don't need IVF to conceive. While PGD can reduce the likelihood of having an affected child, it cannot eliminate the risk. Confirmation with chorionic villus sampling (CVS), amniocentesis, or other testing is still necessary.

Step Five: Transferring the Embryos to the Uterus

The embryos are placed inside the woman's uterus 3 to 5 days after egg collection. The embryologist loads the embryos into a very soft catheter along with a small volume of the culture media in which they are growing. Some clinics, including ours, use EmbryoGlue with each embryo transfer. EmbryoGlue is an implantation-promoting medium for transfer of embryos into the uterus. It has physical properties similar to Mother Nature's own uterine secretion and will therefore assist the embryo during the implantation process.

The physician then inserts the catheter through the cervix and injects the embryos inside the uterine cavity during a speculum examination. The process is similar to an insemination, although it is done under abdominal ultrasound guidance in order to ensure that the catheter is in the proper position to deposit the embryos. No anesthesia is necessary during embryo transfer, although some women may wish to have a mild sedative.

The number of embryos transferred depends upon the age of the patient, the quality of the embryos and the stage of their development. Our clinic follows the guidelines set forth by the Society for Assisted Reproductive Technology (SART) and the American Society for Reproductive Medicine (ASRM). SART's guidelines are geared to maximize a couple's chance of pregnancy while minimizing their chance of having more babies than they would like to have. Since each embryo has a probability of implantation and development, the number of embryos to be placed should be determined specifically for each patient, taking into account the odds of achieving a pregnancy based on the number of embryos transferred and weighing the risk of multiple gestation.

After egg retrieval, patients are given progesterone and estrogen medications to help create a uterine lining that is optimal for embryo implantation. Two weeks after the egg retrieval, a pregnancy test (hCG level) tells us if we were successful. Pregnant patients have a repeat hCG test after 2 days to ensure that the hormone is rising appropriately. An ultrasound study is performed approximately 4 weeks after the egg collection to determine how many fetuses are present and their viability.

Embryo Freezing (*Cryopreservation*)

Some couples are fortunate enough to obtain a large number of embryos from one egg collection. Any viable embryos that are not transferred into the woman's uterus during the month of treatment may be frozen (cryopreserved) in small tubes and kept in storage in the embryo laboratory for future use. This allows the patient to limit the number of embryos transferred "fresh" without sacrificing the chance that the unused embryos could lead to a pregnancy. The embryos may be kept in storage for several years.

By transferring frozen-thawed embryos into the uterus, some patients have achieved two or three pregnancies in different years from just one egg collection. Cryopreservation makes future ART cycles simpler, less expensive, and less invasive than the initial IVF cycle, since the woman does not require ovarian stimulation or egg retrieval. However, not all embryos survive the freezing and thawing process, and the live birth rate is lower with the transfer of cryopreserved embryos. Couples should decide if they are going to cryopreserve extra embryos before undergoing IVF.

Success Rates with In Vitro Fertilization

The most recent rates for individual IVF programs in the United States are available on the Internet from the Society for Assisted Reproductive Technology (SART) at www.sart.org and from the Centers for Disease Control and

Prevention at www.cdc.gov/art. Although this information is readily available, the results should be interpreted carefully.

The success rates of an IVF center depend upon a number of factors, and a comparison of clinic success rates is not meaningful because patient characteristics and treatment approaches vary from clinic to clinic. The type of patients accepted into the program and the numbers of embryos transferred per cycle affect the program's statistics.

Statistics calculated on small numbers of cycles may not be accurate. An IVF center's rates may change dramatically over time, and the compiled statistics may not represent a program's current success. It is also important to understand the definitions of pregnancy rates and live birth rates. For example, a pregnancy rate of 40 percent does not mean that 40 percent of women took babies home. Pregnancy does not always result in live birth. A *biochemical pregnancy* is a pregnancy confirmed by blood or urine tests, but is not visible on ultrasound, because the pregnancy stops developing before it is far enough along. A *clinical pregnancy* is one in which the pregnancy is seen with ultrasound, but stops developing sometime afterward. Therefore, when comparing the pregnancy rates of different clinics, it is important to know which type of pregnancy is being compared.

Most couples, of course, are more concerned with a clinic's live birth rate, which is the proportion of babies delivered to IVF cycle started. Pregnancy rates, and more importantly, birth rates, are influenced by a number of factors, including the woman's age.

CHAPTER THIRTEEN

The Egg Preservation Option

THIS WAS GREGG Henzel's reaction to the birth of his baby son Hayden: "He eats. He sleeps. He cries. He goes to the bathroom. He's awesome," Gregg told a Denver newspaper.

Hayden Henzel was the first baby born in Colorado from a mother's egg that had been frozen and then stored in liquid nitrogen. His parents, Gregg and Carolyn Henzel, had tried to start a family for more than 5 years. They talked to many doctors and experts but their frustrations only grew until we selected Carolyn as one of 13 patients for an experimental procedure, called *vitrification*, to freeze their eggs then quickly thaw them.

Since the use of vitrification began, more than 500 children have been born from frozen eggs. More and more women are choosing this relatively new procedure, which can be a blessing for those who

○ Wish to preserve their fertility for a later time

○ Are facing medical treatments with chemotherapy or radiation that would destroy their eggs

○ Are diagnosed with a systemic disease, such as lupus, rheumatoid arthritis, that may require significant medical therapy

The concept of egg freezing was developed only in the 1980s. Years of successfully freezing sperm motivated scientists to overcome the challenges of freezing eggs, too. In the early days of egg freezing, the process was fraught with difficulties due to the water content of the egg. Early attempts to freeze eggs were thwarted by the fact that the water in the egg formed ice crystals and broke up the egg's cellular machinery, including the chromosomes and spindle complexes that rearrange the chromosomes during cellular division.

When the eggs were thawed, most had suffered irreparable damage. There was a less than a 10 percent survival rate for frozen eggs, and of those that survived less than 10 percent were fertilized, and women using frozen eggs had a pregnancy rate of less than 10 percent. Until recently, only about 200 children had been born to mothers using frozen eggs because of all the complications.

Yet most of those challenges have been overcome in recent years thanks to a revolutionary new technique that completely changed the process of egg freezing. Vitrification is a rapid freezing process in which the egg is protected with cryoprotectants and plunged into liquid nitrogen, which has a temperature of minus 196°C. The freezing process takes about 30 seconds and results in the egg rapidly going from a liquid state to a glass state. It is frozen so fast that the egg doesn't form ice crystals. Once readied, the frozen egg is warmed, also at a rapid rate, to return it to a living, functioning egg.

Hope for the Henzels and countless other couples increased greatly because of vitrification. I visited scientists in Japan and Spain to learn about this method from its pioneers, and then our team helped refine the process.

The survival rate with vitrification has dramatically improved, with more than 80 percent survival, and fertilization rates of more than 80 percent. The pregnancy rate in our pilot study approached 70 percent. These numbers are equivalent to those we achieve with fresh eggs.

Embryos, or fertilized eggs, have been frozen for several decades now, with great success. Because the cells within the embryo are much smaller than the egg cell, the problem of ice crystal formation is not as great. Embryo freezing has resulted in many thousands of pregnancies and is available not only for fertility preservation, but also for surplus embryos after an IVF cycle. The use of vitrification also has greatly improved the survival of embryos. The long-term storage, outcomes, and risks associated with frozen embryos are well documented—these issues remain to be answered with egg vitrification because it is still in its infancy.

Fertility Frozen in Time

The bottom line is that egg vitrification helps preserve your fertility and it gives you the option to pursue pregnancy when you choose to pursue it rather than having your options limited by your biological clock or a medical condition. Thanks to this process, women now have a better chance of getting pregnant with eggs they froze in their thirties than with their own unfrozen eggs in their forties.

Women who wish to have their eggs frozen solely to preserve their fertility are best served to have this procedure when they are young—less than 35 years old is optimal, and they should definitely be less than 40 years old for best results. By freezing your eggs, you effectively stop the biological clock. Whether you choose to use your vitrified eggs shortly after freezing or to wait until you are 45 years old, your eggs will not age beyond the point of their freezing—and your chances of getting pregnant will be based on that same "frozen" age. In effect, you will become your own egg donor.

Denise, 33, came to our clinic after becoming a partner in a prestigious law firm. She was not in a relationship, and she wanted to dedicate another 8 to 10 years to her career before starting a family. Yet Denise also wanted to have her own biological children one day, so, to ensure that her eggs would remain viable, she decided to have them frozen to be used at a later date.

Another patient, a young television news anchor, came to our clinic to discuss her options for having a family one day—but not just yet. She had been hired for a television network news job and her new employer told her that she had to commit to at least 8 years of uninterrupted work.

"I want to be sure that my eggs are not too old by the time I'm able to start my family," she told us.

We told her that freezing her eggs at a young age would give her the opportunity to conceive at a much later age, even well into her forties.

An Option for Women Faced with Cancer

Besides preserving your fertility, this process offers a blessing for reproductive-aged women who must undergo cancer treatment. There are relatively few other options for preserving fertility in women—such as using leuprolide acetate to decrease ovarian function, or removing a piece of the ovary to save for later—have not had high rates of success.

Because you produce only a finite number of eggs, those damaged by either chemotherapy or radiation are lost forever. Yet, with cancer survival rates improving continually, many women want to have children after they recover.

Margie was 31 years old, and engaged to be married when she was diagnosed with colon cancer. Her oncologist advised that she had a few weeks to pursue fertility preservation. Since she wasn't yet married, she didn't want to create embryos. Instead, she decided to preserve her eggs to use after her treatment. If she succumbed to her cancer, she couldn't bear the thought of leaving "children" behind from created embryos. She froze her eggs quickly and then underwent chemotherapy and radiation. We are happy to report that she survived her cancer and is doing well. Happily married, she plans to start a family in a few years with her frozen eggs.

Many single women faced with cancer treatment decide to freeze their eggs instead of creating embryos from a donor sperm, therefore giving them the opportunity to fertilize their eggs with a partner's sperm when they are ready. Women with cancer who are in a relationship can choose to use their partner's sperm and freeze the embryos instead of the eggs.

The key to fertility preservation for the female cancer patient is to consult with an fertility specialist as soon as possible once you are diagnosed. Most women are naturally first concerned about their immediate health and the impact of the cancer on their lives, their families, and their careers. That is understandable, of course. Yet it is important for women of childbearing age to consider their options for starting a family after their cancer treatments have done their job. The process for freezing your eggs requires about 2 weeks for stimulation and retrieval of the eggs. You and your oncologist need to determine that this delay won't compromise your cancer treatment.

Cancer does not discriminate—it affects people of all ages. A woman may or may not have a partner when it strikes. Egg vitrification now offers options where few were present before.

Women with systemic diseases that affect the whole body—such as rheumatoid arthritis, systemic lupus, severe endometriosis, and other significant conditions—should consider this therapy as well. They will often have a longer time to consider the option than those facing cancer treatment. The process remains the same.

An Alternative to Embryo Preservation

Although most women who freeze their eggs do so to preserve their fertility, vitrification has also created opportunities for women who have ethical, religious, or moral objections about creating surplus embryos. During in vitro fertilization, all eggs are typically fertilized to give the best chances of pregnancy and then your doctors select the best embryos, and often couples have extra embryos left over that can be frozen. In the United States, there is a huge surplus of embryos that may never be used.

Hillary and Mark were high school sweethearts and married early. They had struggled with infertility for more than 9 years. After many attempts at pregnancy, they chose to pursue IVF in the days prior to the development of egg vitrification. Hillary was just 28 years old and stimulated very well with medications. She had 32 eggs retrieved and 28 fertilized with Mark's sperm. After transferring two embryos, she had 13 embryos that were frozen—more than she would ever likely need or use. They completed IVF prior to the development of egg freezing, and they wanted to maximize their chances of success, so they fertilized all of the eggs.

Hillary conceived twins and delivered a boy and a girl. This couple wanted just two children, but they still have thirteen more potential lives in the freezer. They feel obligated to these embryos but they do not want more children. Their options for the frozen embryos include discarding them, donating them to research, or donating them to another couple.

Hillary and Mark are still weighing their choices. Had they completed IVF after vitrification was available, they would have had the option of fertilizing some of the eggs while freezing extras to avoid an excess of embryos and the moral dilemma of what to do with them.

Vitrification and Egg Donation

Aside from fertility preservation, egg freezing creates many new possibilities for egg donation. Currently, the majority of eggs from a donor cycle are being received fresh. With egg freezing, a bank of donor eggs could be created to expedite the process and further enhance safety for the recipients by holding the eggs so that the donor can be reassessed for infectious diseases that may be passed to their recipient. The odds of transmitting disease are low with fresh eggs, but could be even lower with frozen eggs.

So far, there does not appear to be any increased chance for birth defects or abnormalities in children born from frozen eggs. There are still questions remaining regarding this technique because it is a fairly new method. As more and more children are conceived from frozen eggs, we will learn more about vitrification's effects. It's also true that we have yet to determine whether there should be limits on how long eggs should remain frozen. We assume, for now, that they can remain frozen in liquid nitrogen forever, but there are not enough cases to know the impact as yet.

Although we assume that all eggs that are mature and frozen will survive, there may be some eggs from some women that do not survive. We won't know more about this until many more women undergo the process.

The Egg Freezing Process

The process for egg freezing is similar to IVF with a few extra steps along the way. First, the eggs are stimulated by injectable medication to make as many grow as possible. Once the eggs reach the right size, they are surgically retrieved and evaluated for maturity. Mature eggs can be frozen for use later. At this time, the process stops until the woman decides to use them.

When the patient is ready to try and start a family, her uterus is prepared for embryo transfer with estrogen and progesterone. The eggs are warmed and then fertilized with sperm via *intracytoplasmic sperm injection* (ICSI). The number of eggs warmed is decided by the patient.

ICSI is necessary because the shell (*zona pellucida*) of the egg become less receptive to sperm after freezing. Without ICSI, the likelihood of fertilization decreases rapidly. The embryos are transferred back to the uterus on either day 3 or day 5. Any extra embryos or eggs are then frozen. (See Chapter 12 on in vitro fertilization for further details.)

Egg-freezing costs range from $9,000 to $15,000 per attempt. There is also an annual storage fee of $350 to $15,000 depending on the location. As costly as it can be, this treatment is helping thousands of women worldwide.

CHAPTER FOURTEEN

The Gestational Surrogacy Option

BECKY WAS A healthy and outgoing 34-year-old who'd enjoyed a successful career and a 6-year marriage. Unfortunately, she had not achieved one major goal: to have a baby. For 2 years, she and her husband, Jeff, tried to conceive without success.

During that time, Becky had lost two early pregnancies. The first was diagnosed at a 12-week ultrasound that found only an empty gestational sac. Her second pregnancy was more hopeful, with a heartbeat detected at 7 weeks, but at 9 weeks, Becky experienced bleeding and cramping. She miscarried at home.

Becky's physician reassured her that her experiences were not uncommon. He said a medical evaluation was only necessary if she had another loss. Hesitant to try again, Becky and Jeff decided to take a few months off and restart their attempt at a family the following fall. They were comforted by friends who shared similar stories of having miscarriages before they finally had children. Becky took heart when she quickly conceived after just a month of trying again that fall. But then she lost the fetus at 10 weeks. She and her physician agreed that a D&C (dilatation and curettage) should be performed to obtain tissue to determine whether a chromosomal abnormality in the fetus caused the miscarriage.

After the surgical procedure, Becky was referred to a reproductive specialist for further testing. Preliminary evaluation for uterine deformities, autoimmune issues, and blood clotting issues turned up nothing out of the ordinary. After 4 weeks, the tests on the fetal chromosomes revealed that it had been a normal male. Becky was frustrated with the lack of answers.

At that point, Becky's only options were to try again or to consider the use of a gestational carrier. Although there was no obvious reason for her continued miscarriages, she continued to miscarry. In this situation, we often use a gestational carrier because the uterus simply isn't working.

Gestational carriers—as distinct from surrogate mothers—agree to carry an implanted embryo from another woman through to delivery. Most people are familiar with traditional surrogacy, also known as compensated or commercial surrogacy, which became popular in the 1980s, but has sometimes been controversial, resulting in custody battles and other legal issues.

In the traditional surrogate mother scenario, the surrogate allows herself to be inseminated with the sperm from the partner of the intended parents. This differs from gestational carriers, who have no biological link to the child. In many states, contractual agreements for traditional surrogacy will not be upheld, as the carrier is both the birth mother and the genetic mother and thus has inalienable legal rights.

Becky opted for a gestational carrier. After working for several months with an agency, she chose a wonderful stay-at-home mother from California who had two children of her own. This woman, Jessica, had an uncomplicated obstetrical history so she appeared to be capable of carrying Becky's child to term.

Jessica signed a contractual agreement with Becky and Jeff. Both women then underwent numerous tests to ensure that the process—in vitro fertilization (IVF)—would be successful. Both were started on birth control pills to synchronize their cycles. Jessica started estrogen patches to allow appropriate development of her lining, while Becky began daily injections to induce multiple follicular development.

As the time of egg retrieval approached, Becky began having some doubts. She said she was terrified that this would not work. Jessica and Jeff were very understanding and supportive. As often happens, Jessica became a friend to Becky and a constant source of encouragement.

Becky continued with the plan. She stimulated well, with 21 eggs retrieved and 18 fertilized. Of these, 9 were cultured and developed into high-grade blastocysts, each having 60 to 100 cells. The two best embryos were transferred into Jessica's uterus with Becky and Jeff at her side. Each embryo had a central cavity that was expanded and tightly compacted cells that lined the cavity, which would eventually develop into the placenta. Within each cavity, a cluster of cells could be distinctly seen. This would develop into the fetus and eventually a baby.

Two weeks later, Jessica heard the good news. She quickly called Becky. The first of many hurdles had been overcome. The embryos had implanted in Jessica's uterus. The next hurdle would be the ultrasound. At exactly 5 weeks after the retrieval, an ultrasound was performed on Jessica at the clinic. We confirmed two gestational sacs, each with a fetus and a fluttering heartbeat.

At Becky's insistence, weekly ultrasounds were performed until 11 weeks. They were all promising and reassuring. Jessica delivered at 35 weeks, a healthy boy and a healthy girl.

While a great deal of modern technology was applied in the delivery of Becky's twins, the concept of surrogacy dates back to antiquity. In the book of Genesis, Sarah asks Hagar, her Egyptian handmaiden, to carry a child for her and Abraham.

In the 1970s, the first brokered legal agreement was made between a set of intended parents and a traditional surrogate for no compensation. In 1980, the first documented commercial surrogacy contract was arranged, for $10,000. The birth mother in that case eventually regretted her decision and is now an advocate against traditional surrogacy.

In 1985, the first gestational surrogacy in the United States was performed for a couple in which the wife had undergone a hysterectomy. A year later, the infamous case of Baby M was center stage of most news stories. The traditional surrogate mother, Mary Beth Whitehead, gave birth to Baby M and decided that she wanted custody. What ensued was a 2-year court battle, with the intended parents getting custody but the surrogate mother getting visitation rights.

Due to these legal challenges, some states have adopted strict legislation that either does not recognize contractual agreements or prohibits them. Some states have either no provisions against surrogacy or have ruled in favor of cases concerning surrogacy agreements. In addition, some state laws hold that such agreements can only be made between the surrogate and a married couple.

Any couples or individuals who proceed down this path must have legal counsel, and they should do their research so they understand the laws pertaining to surrogacy in their state. The legal challenges to traditional surrogacy are so great in many parts of the country that surrogate mothers have been abandoned and replaced by gestational carriers.

Who might be interested in a gestational carrier? Most of our patients who choose this path are women who have undergone hysterectomies (for cancers, for example, or for bleeding complications at the time of birth) or women who have uterine deformities, complicated obstetrical histories, multiple failed IVF cycles, or other medical conditions that have prevented them from carrying their own babies to successful delivery.

Single men and gay partners can also use gestational carriers, depending on the law in the state where their gestational carrier will deliver the baby. The legal aspect becomes even more precarious when a party is not genetically related to the child; for example, if an embryo is produced from donor sperm and donor eggs, or if they choose a donated embryo. State laws vary in those situations. In some states, the gestational carrier may be granted custody or visitation rights.

For international patients from countries that have prohibited the use of gestational carriers, it is important to investigate the necessary legal steps for obtaining passports for the infant to return home with the parents. In addition, most agencies charge additional fees to coordinate care.

I recommend using gestational carriers only if there is an obstetrical or medical need for this option. Even if someone voluntarily and contractually agrees to carry the baby or babies of intended parents, there are risks to the carrier's health and even her life that make it unacceptable and unethical to use this method merely for convenience or vanity.

Beginning the Process
of Using a Gestational Carrier

Most patients consult with an infertility clinic to initiate care. Due to the complexity and legal aspects, clinics rarely provide gestational carriers. Patients are referred to agencies in the United States. These agencies recruit carriers and are often run by attorneys, former medical professionals such as nurses, or individuals who have served as gestational carriers themselves. They are responsible for doing criminal and financial background checks on each candidate. Those with financial difficulties, such as liens on a home or property, and anyone on state assistance programs are unsuitable candidates because of concern that they might be offering the service solely to make money.

The agency should do a preliminary screen of the gestational carrier's medical history, but this does not guarantee the person you choose will clear a clinic's medical and obstetrical requirements, which are often more stringent. The agency also should assist in coordinating the legal work and provide counseling support for the gestational carrier before, during, and after the process.

Most important, the fees paid to the agency and the gestational carrier should be placed in a legitimate escrow account for the protection of all parties. The agency should not have the ability to withdraw any money from the escrow account. Be aware that these agencies are not regulated, so it is of the utmost importance that intended parents verify the legitimacy of the services that are to be provided. You also should make certain that the agency and its escrow account are insured.

Unfortunately, there have been reports of unscrupulous agencies that have taken money from aspiring parents but never provided the services they'd promised. Don't be discouraged. There are several outstanding agencies throughout the United States that provide wonderful services to intended parents. The main point is to be careful. Do your homework and investigate the agency, the attorneys, and the escrow company.

A list of our customary charges for gestational carriers follows. The fees including IVF charges, are typically $70,000 to $90,000. In cases where the insurance of the gestational carrier excludes surrogacy, you will need to purchase a health policy that may run as high as $20,000.

USING A GESTATIONAL CARRIER

SURROGATE SERVICES	APPROXIMATE COSTS
Agency fee	$18,000–25,000
Psychological fees	$4,200
Legal fees	$3,500–$5,600
Surrogate fees	$24,000
Variable costs	$2,000–$5,000
Medical costs	TBD

The fees for professional gestational carriers are out of range for many couples. Some may turn to friends or family members for their gestational carriers, who will still need to meet the stringent medical and legal guidelines used for agency carriers.

We've also known aspiring parents who have turned to the Internet in search of a more affordable gestational carrier. Intended parents and gestational carriers who for whatever reasons prefer to work directly with each other, without the assistance of an agency, often search blogs or list their needs or services on Craigslist.org and similar Web sites. Some wonderful relationships have developed from such sources, but we advise you to be very cautious in taking this route, as some couples have been taken advantage of. There are predators and unscrupulous people in every line of business, and gestational carriers are no exception.

Aside from legal considerations, gestational carriers must meet a number of important criteria. She must have delivered and be raising at least one child, and have a pregnancy history that's free of complications. She must be a non-smoker between the ages of 21 and 40 with a body mass index between 18 and 30. She should enjoy being pregnant and live in a safe and stable environment. Candidates with a criminal history or who are living on government assistance will not be approved.

Once a binding legal contract has been drawn and she has met the general profile, the gestational carrier will need to undergo thorough medical and psychological testing to ensure she is a suitable candidate. Her previous medical and obstetrical records will be reviewed. She will meet with a physician for a thorough physical and pelvic exam as well as an ultrasound to ensure the uterus is normal. The clinic's physicians will evaluate the gestational carrier's uterine cavity with an office hysteroscopy or saline ultrasound. The gestational carrier also will have extensive infectious disease testing. Her husband or partner will need to undergo the same testing to ensure that he has no infections that might be transmitted to the baby.

The gestational carrier as well as her husband or partner will be required to meet with a trained counselor or psychologist for evaluation. A personality inventory test will be administered and if there is any concern regarding the carrier's psychological well-being, she will not be approved as a gestational carrier.

Working with Your Gestational Carrier

Once your candidate gestational carrier has been evaluated and approved and has signed all legal documents, you both will start taking Lupron to prevent ovulation. You will begin taking gonadotropins to stimulate multiple follicular development, allowing us to harvest several eggs at one time. During this stage, the gestational carrier is preparing her endometrium with estrogen.

When your eggs are to be retrieved, the gestational carrier will begin progesterone support, either as intramuscular injections or with vaginal suppositories that recently received FDA approval for luteal support in IVF cycles.

After the eggs are fertilized, the embryos are grown in the laboratory for 3 to 5 days. If you are 40 or over, 3 to 4 embryos may be transferred to compensate for the lower implantation rates associated with genetic abnormalities that increase with a woman's age. At our clinic, birth rates have been documented as high as 70 percent, but will be lower in women 41 or older. In cases where an egg donor is used, the delivery rates have been in the 80 percent range.

Depending on state laws, a birth order may be obtained to place your and your partner's name on the birth certificate, and in other states adoption proceedings may be required. Remember, the state in which the carrier delivers is where the attorneys for both parties must be practicing.

The number of aspiring parents using gestational carriers increases each year as this option becomes more widely accepted. It is indeed a viable option for patients who have had hysterectomies or for women who cannot carry a pregnancy for other medical reasons.

Our patient Ericka chose this option after being diagnosed with a T-shaped uterus. Many women with this condition are able to conceive, but unfortunately many give birth prematurely. She and her husband, Jason, used a surrogacy agency based in Houston.

"My biggest stress was giving up total control—control of the pregnancy to another person. When you work with a surrogacy agency, one of the requirements of the surrogates is that they already have at least one child of their own. It terrified me that I was asking someone's mom to carry my baby for me. I was terrified that something could go wrong and leave another family without a mother," Ericka said.

The matching process with Ericka's surrogacy agency seemed like an "arranged marriage" at first, and their first encounter with surrogate Rebecca and her husband, Mike, was "surreal," she said.

"I knew right away that we had found the right person. It took Jason all of 5 minutes to decide to work with them, too.

"Our initial impressions proved correct. We had a great experience with them," Ericka said.

The next 3 months flew by. Once they completed the required medical and legal documentation, Rebecca and Ericka began their shots for the IVF process.

"There were many things I wish I'd known going into the medical procedures. One of those was the fact that egg retrieval is not a guaranteed success. While I had eighteen eggs retrieved, only nine were mature. I did not know that some would be immature. I thought that if you retrieved an egg it was automatically good to go," she said.

Only 5 of the 9 eggs resulted in an embryo. Of the 5 embryos, only 3 survived. Two embryos were transferred in Rebecca's uterus on day 3. About 10 days later, Rebecca called to say she might be pregnant. The official test confirmed the positive pregnancy a few days later. Now came a long, 4-week wait until the first ultrasound at week 6.

Sadly, the smaller of the babies died sometime before the week 8 ultrasound, but the larger baby continued to grow normally. The rest of Rebecca's pregnancy proceeded without incident except for a minor bleeding scare at week 10.

Rebecca delivered baby Jacob 4 weeks early, but he weighed a very healthy 5 pounds, 3 ounces, and measured 17.5 inches. Because he was premature, his lungs were not fully developed, so he had to stay in the neonatal intensive care unit for 2 weeks until his lungs were ready for the world. But Jacob has been a healthy, rambunctious young man who has made his parents very happy that they went through this often arduous but ultimately rewarding process.

CHAPTER FIFTEEN

Alternative Treatments for Infertility

CATHY, 40, HAD tried everything within her power to get pregnant before she came to us for treatment. She'd been through a long series of tests and treatments at another clinic, including four in vitro fertilization (IVF) procedures.

She and her husband had a number of infertility challenges. Her husband's sperm count was low but marginally acceptable. She had unexplained hormonal imbalances. At one point, Cathy was diagnosed with unexplained fertility. She later was found to have poor-quality eggs.

Cathy was discouraged with Western medicine's failure to help her conceive. Fortunately, she found Randine Lewis, an expert in alternative approaches to fertility treatment. Randine is the founder of the Fertile Soul, a body, mind, and spirit program and institute and Web site (www.thefertilesoul.com). She is a licensed acupuncturist and herbalist who began her studies in Western medicine, then focused on Eastern medicine and its methods for treating infertility after she had trouble getting pregnant.

Randine, who at the time Cathy saw her had an alternative medicine clinic in Houston, gave Cathy herbs, herbal teas, and acupuncture treatments to "restore the balance" of her body and reproductive system and to help reduce her high level of stress. After Randine's treatments, Cathy began to feel much healthier, but still, she did not become pregnant. Yet she had the sense that physically and mentally she was in a better place.

Finally, Cathy decided to try in vitro fertilization one more time. Randine gave her blessing and suggested Cathy contact our clinic. We often get referrals from Randine Lewis, and we also refer patients to her if they are willing to try a combination of alternative and conventional approaches. That was the case with Cathy. When she came to us after taking Randine's treatments, we told her that although her medical history suggested another IVF would not work, we were willing to try if she was.

We encouraged her to continue with Randine's treatments while we treated her, too. While there is not always a scientific explanation for Randine's alternative methods, we've found them to be beneficial to the health of our patients.

Cathy went through an IVF cycle at our clinic while also taking herbs and other treatments from Randine. All of us were delighted when her IVF cycle succeeded, she became pregnant, and she delivered a healthy child.

When it comes to Randine's Eastern medical approaches, there are just some things I can't explain, but they seem to be beneficial, so I try to keep an open mind. Alternative, or *complementary*, medicine, as it is sometimes known, is something I cannot ignore as an infertility physician whose priority is helping his patients achieve their dreams of having children.

Approximately half of my patients have already tried some form of unconventional therapy before they come to our clinic. Most patients at some point seek any and all methods for improving their chances of having a child. I share with my patients every safe and healthy method I know, whether Eastern or Western, that might be helpful. Chinese herbs and acupuncture are the most common of these alternative therapies. I can't say that I have mastered the science, but acupuncture has in fact been shown to improve ovulation and pregnancy rates in patients with polycystic ovary syndrome.

Acupuncture affects B-endorphin levels in the central nervous system, which in turn affect the hormones that control ovulation. So there is some clinical basis to such treatment. Acupuncture has also been studied as a method of pain relief for egg retrieval and as a means of increasing pregnancy rates with IVF. Acupuncture on the day of embryo transfer appears to affect uterine blood flow and the frequency of uterine contractions. Both of these mechanisms theoretically improve the ability of the uterus to accept embryos. Indeed, a meta-analysis (a summary of the medical studies) has shown an improvement in IVF outcome with the addition of acupuncture.

I am no expert on Chinese medicine or other unconventional or folk medicines, but I often refer patients to Randine Lewis when they express an interest in treatments from the East. I have included information from her in this chapter so that you will have an overview of this field. You can then decide if this is something you want to use to augment your Western-medicine approach to infertility. I am thankful to Randine for sharing her expertise with us.

Randine and other advocates of Eastern medicine don't like to use the term *alternative* because they consider these approaches to be natural modes of healing that are complementary to Western medicine. Sometimes, as happened in Cathy's case, patients who receive a bit of nature's remedies from Eastern medicine become more responsive to the science of Western medical treatments.

East Meets West

Did you have earaches as a child? Many children remember their mothers placing a hot, wet cloth over their ears to "steam" them, reducing the pain from internal pressure. Often, that was all it took to relieve the pain, but sometimes an antibiotic was needed to complete the job. The pill and the hot cloth worked together to give more relief than either would have done alone. Randine and I approach our combining of Eastern and Western medicine in much the same way when we treat fertility patients open to these techniques. I handle West. She does East.

Just because conception hasn't happened naturally doesn't mean that Eastern medicine's natural methods won't improve the patient's response. Every assisted reproductive method holds a better chance of success when the patient can support it by improving their overall reproductive health. Once a patient has improved her inherent reproductive capacity, she tends to respond better to intervention, and she also bounces back more quickly after unsuccessful treatments because she is simply better equipped—physically, mentally, emotionally, and spiritually.

Proven over thousands of years in Asia, and especially in China, the Eastern approach to infertility has been responsible for millions of births. Chinese methods have only recently been widely studied by practitioners of Western reproductive medicine, and many have found these methods improve fertility.

Acupuncture in particular has been scientifically shown to enhance fertility by balancing hormones and increasing blood flow to the pelvic organs, thereby reducing the physiologic response to stress.

Of course, acupuncture has been used for centuries in Asian cultures to enhance fertility. But more and more doctors in the United States and Europe have been using acupuncture to improve reproductive functions in their patients. I will familiarize you with some other ways Chinese medicine has been found to improve your fertility.

Traditions of Eastern Medicine

According to ancient Chinese philosophy, all life comes from a source of energy called the *Tao*. Just as one cell begins the process of human life, this wholeness or oneness runs throughout nature. The Chinese believe that Tao is responsible for all of life and is manifest in energetic patterns of interaction. But all parts retain the memory of oneness.

Randine says that fertility recognizes this power of wholeness. In this context, fertility is not seen as a mere product of the reproductive organs, but as a complex interaction of the whole, involving our environment and the biology of our bodies, down to our hormones and the interaction of the egg and the sperm.

Yin and Yang

Some of the following material may sound a bit unusual to you, but this form of medicine has been practiced for thousands of years. While modern science may not always be able to explain why and how these methods work, they have been effective for many people over the generations.

In Asian culture, it is believed that the spirit underlying all existence separates into two divisions, known as *yin* (the feminine, receptive energy), and *yang* (the masculine, active energy.) The first energetic division is responsible for all of life, from heaven and earth on down to the positive and negative charges in an atom. The second, yang, represents the spark of life, heat, and the body's ability to generate and maintain warmth and circulation.

In reproductive terms, yin is the egg and yang is the sperm. Together they cause a fertilized zygote to divide into two cells, then four, then eight, and so on until the result is a fully formed human being.

Eastern medicine is all about maintaining a balance between the yin and the yang. In Eastern fertility treatments, it is believed that three elements are manifest in the human body to bring forth conditions necessary for a baby to grow: *jing* (essence), *qi* (energy), and *shen* (spirit), manifested as body, mind, and spirit, respectively. Just as the sun can be said to be hot, bright, and powerful, these three elements cannot be separated from each other; they are three ways of looking at the one.

Advocates of Eastern medicine believe that the germinating essence of life (the body) is what makes up the womb, the egg, and the sperm. The mind provides the interactive energies (thoughts and emotions) that determine how hormones are produced, distributed, and received; the spirit of the internal sun, allowing implantation and emergence, comes from the ultimate internal source of healing, the heart.

Yin, Yang, Qi, and Blood

In Eastern medicine, it is believed that during the growth of the embryo there is an inner alignment that differentiates the baby in progress into specific developmental patterns that govern the earliest embryonic period. These are supported by the balanced interaction of yin (supports estrogen production and follicular growth), yang (supports progesterone production and luteal phase support), qi (manifested by ovulation and hormone metabolism), and menstrual blood.

Practitioners of Eastern medicine hold that when yin is weak or obstructed, often estrogen levels are abnormal and the follicular phase may malfunction. When yang is weak, often women can't sustain the luteal phase.

When qi is insufficient or obstructed, ovulation or the premenstrual transition are not smooth. And when menstrual blood is deficient or blocked, the menstruation itself will be problematic.

Chinese Medicine:
Water, Wood, Earth, Metal, and Fire

The Eastern tradition, like many ancient cultures around the world, holds that five major elements—water, wood, earth, metal, and fire—are the catalysts for creation. Chinese practitioners focus on harmonizing these elements to create a healthy life. Western medicine uses similar systemic maps, but they are broken down into an anatomic system, whereas Chinese medicine pays more attention to energy relationships. In a nutshell, these elements and their Western correlations are:

○ Water—reproductive organs, genetic contribution from germ cells

○ Wood—the liver's ability to metabolize and release hormones

○ Earth—contents of digestion, metabolism, and nutritional distribution

○ Metal—creation of the physical structure that becomes the breath of life

○ Fire—the spirit of existence, located in the heart and brain chemistry

According to practitioners of Chinese medicine, when any of these energetic systems is thrown out of balance—either by external disease, internal emotional disturbance, or living out of harmony with nature's law—infertility can result. These patterns of imbalance result from either deficiencies or excesses. Deficient patterns are often seen when hormone levels are low, gonadal output is diminished, or the uterus responds weakly. Excess patterns are often represented by obstructed energies that can result from certain high levels of hormones, conditions like polycystic ovary syndrome, blocked tubes, or obstructed uterine conditions like endometriosis or fibroids.

Creating Balance

When we can create an environment of balance, life is manifest on its own, according to Eastern medicine. We don't need to force it. Watch buds emerging in the springtime—when conditions are right, life comes on its own.

On the other hand, as you know if you have ever nurtured a seed into a plant, no amount of coaxing or fertilizing is going to make the little seedling pop out of the ground.

Many infertility patients worry so much about their fertility that they seem to counter it. Often, stress and a hectic lifestyle are not conducive to life coming on its own, so you may need some help finding balance. Chinese medicine associates fertility with the fertile valley rather than the mountain peak. It takes effort to reach the peak, and we've all been conditioned to achieve our goals through effort. Climbing to the top of the mountain may land you great jobs and money, but it defies the laws of nature as far as reproduction.

The top of the peak is barren and lifeless. Fertility resides in the valley. Yet many patients are determined to keep pushing up the hill. To achieve fertility, you must follow the natural flow, like that of a stream descending into a valley, according to the Eastern traditions.

Our entire reproductive system is, in fact, based upon receptivity, which is a valley, or yin concept. Hormones activate the cells by fitting into cell receptors. When the body is in the yang mode, struggling to reach a goal, the cell's receptors effectively close down in response to our stressful effort, and the cells can't respond to the hormonal messages very well.

In turn, yang hormones are released from the adrenal glands to help us reach an external goal, making the internal environment even less receptive. Now the body turns its energetic attention *away* from the ovaries and uterus and toward survival functions like beating our heart, activating large muscle groups, and turning our awareness toward our external environment.

Into the Valley

Most of us need a little encouragement to exercise our inherent receptivity. It's already there, and in reality needs no practice; but many of us need to reduce an imbalanced yang activity in order to express our inherent yin nature.

So, how do we become more "valley-like"? Every form of energy has yin and yang components. Both are necessary. Balance is key.

YIN (FERTILE VALLEY)	YANG (MOUNTAIN PEAK)
Rest	Activity
Dark	Light
Internal	External
Estrogen	Follicle-stimulating hormone (FSH)
Uterine lining	Shedding of the lining
Acceptance	Trying to force change

No matter how stressful, or "yang," our lives appear, we can redirect our body's attention away from external details and back toward the internal, fertile valley. It is well understood in all forms of healing and medicine that the more attention we pay to any part of the body, the better it responds.

The following treatments and exercises are presented according to the five elements water, wood, earth, metal, and fire. They direct the body's energies to replenish the reproductive organs, nourishing them with more blood flow, oxygenation, nutrition, and energy, necessary components for fostering healthy eggs and uterine lining. They also reduce the physiologic response to stress, increase delivery of nutrition to all of the cells, and open up the body to life itself.

Balancing the Five Elements for Better Fertility

Water: Reproductive Organs, Genetic Contribution from Germ Cells

The fertile valley is represented by water, like a river flowing through the valley, nourishing all of life. In the body, the water energies are most abundant in the pelvic valley, housing the uterus, ovaries, and fallopian tubes.

Treatment: Femoral Massage, Uterine and Ovarian Massage

This exercise (see Figure 1) can be performed alone or with a partner two times a day before ovulation. Repeat the exercise up to three times. The intention is to increase blood supply to ovaries and uterus.

1. Find the crease between your upper thigh and the trunk of your body (the panty crease).

2. Using your fingertips, locate the femoral artery (as in picture), usually found about one-half to two-thirds of the way in from the outer thigh.

3. Find the pulsation and press down deeply into the artery until you feel the pulse stop at your fingertips.

4. Hold for 30 to 45 seconds and allow the blood flow to gather in the uterus and ovaries.

5. Release the pressure and resume natural flow. You will feel a warm rush as the blood returns down your leg.

6. Repeat on the opposite side.

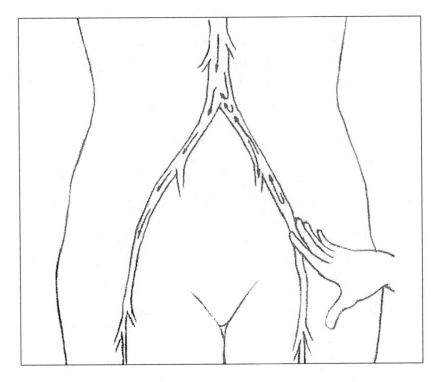

Figure 1: Femoral massage

I recommend performing this exercise three times on each side, twice per day, between the end of your period and ovulation. Do not perform if you have hypertension or glaucoma or if you might be pregnant.

Gently massage the entire lower belly in large clockwise rotations to increase circulation and the overall attention your body pays to this region. When a woman becomes pregnant, where do her hands tend to go automatically? Right to this spot, because her hands seek to connect with the source of life within. The uterus is found about midway between your pubic bone and your navel. Start by bringing your fingers down toward the pubic bone and lift upwards toward the belly button.

Ren 4 (Origin of the Source of the Conception Vessel). Located on the midline, 3 inches below the navel. This point represents the source of life, the center of gravity (*dan tien*) for the body and the site of the uterus. It fortifies the original qi (the life force you inherit from your parents), nourishes kidney essence, and assists conception. Massage with deep, circular motions, but only between menstruation and ovulation. You may also use light, heat, or magnet therapy.

Zigong (Palace of the Child). Located 4 inches below the navel and 3 inches lateral to the midline, (usually just inside the hipbones), this point most closely represents the ovaries. Although you won't be able to feel the ovaries themselves, deep rotational movements increase circulation to the ovarian bed.

Soothing Foot Soak and Other Remedies

A great classic Chinese remedy is a nightly foot soak to improve blood flow to the lower extremities (via the iliac artery through the groin, the same blood supply used by the uterus and ovaries). Fill a basin with warm water. You may add Epsom salts, soothing lavender oil, or invigorating peppermint oil. Submerge your feet and ankles into the warm water. Soak your feet while relaxing to soft music, reading an enjoyable book, or just resting. Breathe deeply into your lower abdomen.

The following acupressure points may be stimulated through circular massage, either with your fingers or other massage devices, or with laser light therapy or magnets.

Ki 3 (Great Ravine). Sometimes an arterial pulsing can be felt at this energetic point, located in the depression behind the inner anklebone and in front of the Achilles tendon, just above the heel bone. This "great ravine," as Ki 3 is also called, nourishes the essence of the reproductive energies. The Great Ravine clears heat that arises because of a deficiency of kidney yin energies.

Ki 7 (Recover the Current). The seventh point of the kidney channel is located 2 inches above the depression behind the inner anklebone, behind the inner leg bone, just on the front border of the Achilles tendon. Ki 7 is the main point of the kidney meridian that tonifies the yang of the kidney. This point also controls whole-body sweating, treats lumbar soreness, resolves dampness in the lower body, and treats kidney yang–deficient diarrhea.

Wood: The Liver's Ability to Metabolize and Release Hormones

Herbs which stimulate ovarian function include Helonias or false unicorn root, Vitex or Chaste tree berry, Epimedium or horny goat weed, and Eucomia. I do not recommend that you take herbs during a stimulated or IVF cycle. I also recommend that all herbs be prescribed by a licensed Chinese herbalist who works closely with a reproductive medicine specialist.

Watch how your body responds to herbs. They generally will not help if your FSH is high, your cycles are short, your estrogen is low, your periods are short, and cervical fluid is scanty. In such cases, you may benefit from Dang Gui or Angelica, or an individually prescribed Kidney Yin tonic.

In Western and Eastern medicine it is well understood that most disease processes, including infertility, are either directly caused by or greatly exacerbated by stress—the inner tension resulting from resisting what is. When we resist and stress out over what is happening in our lives, the hypothalamus translates this message as, "Something's wrong."

As such, beta endorphins and *gonadotropin-releasing hormone* (GnRH), which turns on the reproductive functioning, are released in lower amounts during the perceived stress. This message is also sent to the pituitary gland and switches the body's attention from the ovaries to the adrenal glands, where stress hormones are produced to shift the body's attention *away* from reproductive mode and toward fight-or-flight mode.

We encourage a state of acceptance and nonresistance (not struggling or fighting), which allows the body to shift back into reproductive mode. Practitioners of Eastern medicine believe that sometimes patients need to be detoxed from the accumulated debris of internal stress hormones, not to mention the debris that comes from the coffee, sugars, fat, preservatives, and junk foods they may consume. Over-the-counter medications accumulate in the body, as do the byproducts of alcohol and tobacco. And if a patient has been on any type of external hormone or injectable ovarian stimulation, the liver may become overloaded, and unable to tend to its duties of producing, releasing, and metabolizing new proteins, hormones, and internal chemicals.

Randine recommends occasional 5-day detox plans—not when you are actively trying to conceive, but during your period or a "down" cycle. Eat a diet consisting mostly of colorful, organic, naturally grown produce—vegetables, fruit, beans, and legumes. Leafy green vegetables contain diindolylmethane, or DIM, a chemical that helps your body release excess hormones. Sprouted beans, legumes, and grains are easier on the digestion than those in their seed form. Rice is suitable for a detox plan, as are herbal tea and vegetable broth, although most of your liquid should be in the form of filtered water. Do not worry about an absence of animal products for 5 days. Our bodies are made to receive protein from plant sources. Wheatgrass shots can aid in the detoxification process. Drink milk thistle tea throughout the day to aid the liver-cleansing process. If your intestines need an occasional boost to release stored contents, psyllium husks are a great bulk laxative. Rhubarb root will help expel contents.

Protecting Reproduction

A good defense is the best offense, even in Eastern medicine. By being mindful of physical and emotional stress, you can protect and even improve your reproductive capabilities.

Do not use a laptop on the lap or cell phone worn at the waist. Recent studies have shown that these can have a negative impact on sperm production. Avoid tight underwear, hot tubs, and excessive bike-riding, all which increase scrotal temperature and can reduce sperm counts.

Avoid soy products and foods stored in plastic containers (plasticizers contain a harmful form of synthetic estrogen).

Stress Relief Methods

○ Take a walk in nature

○ Soak in a warm Epsom salt bath with lavender or peppermint oil

○ Listen to soothing music

○ Occasionally indulge in your favorite food or drink—without guilt

○ Receive a whole body massage or foot rub

○ Practice deep belly breathing

○ Try Tai qi, Qi Gong, or yoga classes

○ Allow yourself to experience and safely release whatever emotion comes up

The following acupressure points clear liver energies and reduce the physiologic response to stress.

LI 4 (Joining Valley). Found on the muscular area on the back of the hand about 1 inch inside the web between the base of the thumb and the index finger. LI 4 is often used with Lv 3 (see below) to open up all the channels in the body. Joining Valley alleviates pain and is very effective at resolving premenstrual headaches. It has been found to moderate chemicals responsible for uterine contraction in order to calm the uterus prior to implantation. Acupressure should be used on LI 4 only before ovulation and never during pregnancy. If used during pregnancy, this point can stimulate uterine contractions.

Lv 3 (Great Rushing). Located about 1½ to 2 inches from to the web between the first and second toes, where the point is tender. This point promotes the smooth flow of liver energy, nourishes the liver blood, and treats premenstrual breast pain, headache, depression, and mood swings. Lv 3 is often used in conjunction with LI 4 to open and activate the body's meridians. This combination of points is called the Four Gates. Great Rushing is an important point for regulating menstruation and resolving dysmenorrhea due to stagnant liver energies. This point also has some indications for treating low sperm counts in men with the same pattern.

Lv 14 (Cycle Gate). Cycle Gate is located on the chest approximately 4 inches from the midline in the sixth intercostal space, two ribs below and on the same vertical line as the nipple. Cycle Gate is an important point for resolving stagnant liver qi, especially when it invades the stomach, causing gastrointestinal upset. Lv 14 is helpful in resolving premenstrual breast tenderness, breast pain, and menstrual chills and fevers. Lv 14 allows an opening and relaxation for women who have a tense or uneasy experience with sex. Stimulation of Lv 14 will help a woman become more sexually receptive.

Tai Yang (Greater Yang). Found at the temples, in the depression behind the midpoint between the outside of the eye and eyebrow, this point helps resolve temporal stress headaches and TMJ symptoms.

Earth: Contents of Digestion, Metabolism and Nutritional Distribution

Our digestion, metabolism, and nutritional distribution systems govern the way what we eat is transformed into energy. Having a clean diet allows your body to more efficiently devote its energy to the reproductive process. You are what you eat.

The earth energies govern that which we take in through the diet and transform it into usable energy.

The Asian Diet for Reproductive Health

1. Model your meals on an Asian diet—visualize a plate filled with mostly steamed vegetables, some whole grains, and hand-sized portions of protein.

2. Chew food slowly and mindfully. For optimal digestion, avoid drinking at mealtime and 30 minutes before and after your meal.

3. Eat organic foods, especially if you consume meat or animal products. Leafy greens help the body metabolize excess hormones. Stay away from processed foods.

4. To stabilize blood-sugar levels throughout the day, consume a protein and carbohydrate at each meal and snack. Eliminate all refined sugars and artificial sweeteners. Use low-glycemic natural replacements sparingly (for example, agave nectar, Stevia, xylitol).

5. Replace cow-based dairy products with rice milk, almond milk, or whole-fat sheep's or goat's milk. Cow's milk contains the protein casein, which traditional Chinese medicine considers cloying and dampening. We simply aren't equipped with the enzymes to digest and utilize it properly.

6. Eliminate refined carbohydrates and wheat. Look for sprouted breads (for example, Ezekiel, Food for Life) and products made with spelt flour, rice flour, oat flour, corn flour, and polenta. Choose brown rice over white rice. Use pasta alternatives including spelt, brown rice, spaghetti squash, and quinoa.

7. If you cook with oil, use unrefined organic oils: extra virgin olive oil, sesame oil, peanut oil, and high oleic sunflower oil. Coconut oil is a good choice for recipes that call for very high-temperature cooking.

8. Replace coffee (caffeinated and decaffeinated) with any of the vast array of healing teas: chamomile (calming), ginger (warming, supportive of digestion), red clover (believed to enhance fertility), and peppermint (cooling).

9. If you have heat in the system—short cycles, hot flashes, night sweats—stay away from hot, spicy foods.

10. If your system tends toward being colder, avoid ice-cold drinks and raw, cold foods.

Special Dietary Programs and Nutritional Supplements

Nutritional supplements and special attention to one's diet can help alleviate certain reproductive disorders. What follows is a list of disorders along with supplement regimens and diets that may help treat them.

Polycystic Ovary Syndrome Guidelines

Reduce consumption of sugar, refined carbohydrates, and all nonfat and low fat dairy products.

Supplements that stabilize blood-sugar levels include:

○ Chlorophyll

○ Inositol

○ NAC (N-acetyl cysteine)

○ Chromium picolinate

○ Bitter melon

○ Fenugreek

○ ALA (alpha lipoic acid) (sensitizes cells to insulin, helps liver detox)

○ Saw palmetto (reduces excess testosterone, undermines LH)

Endometriosis Guidelines

Reduce consumption of red meat and all hormonally treated animal products, including dairy. Supplements which help reduce the internal inflammatory reaction to the endometrial cells include:

○ A full complement of antioxidants (vitamins C, E, and B_{12}, beta carotene, and the minerals zinc and selenium)

○ OPC (oligomeric proanthocyanidins)

○ Fish oil, evening primrose oil, flaxseed oil

○ Castor oil (with frankincense essential oils), applied topically with lower abdominal massage

Guidelines for Immunologic Issues

○ No sugar, wheat, or dairy, and reduce all gluten-containing grains

○ Glutathione for gluten sensitivity

- Supplements as listed for endometriosis
- Wobenzym and Nattokinase or Vitalzym Extra Strength, between meals
- Baby aspirin
- PABA along with B vitamins and at least 1000 micrograms of folic acid

Guidelines for Advanced Maternal Age, Poor Ovarian Response, and Poor Egg Quality

- Wheatgrass juice
- Royal jelly
- Co-enzyme Q10
- DHEA and L-arginine can be used for low ovarian reserve (avoid if you have heat signs, such as short cycles, elevated temperatures, acne, hot flashes, and night sweats)

Guidelines for Low Sperm Count

- A full complement of antioxidants (Vitamins C, E, and B_{12}, beta carotene, and the minerals zinc and selenium)
- Amino acids L-arginine and L-carnitine
- Co-enzyme Q10
- Fish oil supplements
- OPC (oligomeric proanthocyanidins) (for poor morphology)
- Ginseng (do not take ginseng if you have a history of high blood pressure)
- Cornus (for poor motility)

The following acupressure points can improve the spleen and digestive energies that support the reproductive process.

St 36 (Lower Sea of Qi). You find this point by holding your leg straight and measuring one handbreadth or 3 inches below the kneecap at the top of the fleshy musculature, 1 inch to the outer side of the crest of the upper shinbone. This name of point is also translated as "3-mile walking," which refers to its effect of strongly tonifying energies, allowing the patient to walk 3 more miles after its stimulation. St 36 tones the qi, fortifies the spleen, nourishes the blood and yin, strengthens resistance, and treats gastrointestinal disorders. Although primarily a spleen and stomach tonic, St 36 tones the qi to help the kidney yang.

Pc 6 (Inner Pass). Located on the inner wrist, about 2 inches proximal to the wrist crease in the depression between the two tendons, Inner Pass (often used in conjunction with Sp 4 to activate the channel between the heart and womb) rectifies the qi and regulates menstruation, calms the mind, and treats anxiety, insomnia, irritability, and the emotional manifestations of premenstrual tension. Pc 6 is also useful in treating symptoms of chest tightness. Often stimulated prior to IVF transfer, Pc 6 opens the heart.

Sp 4 (Grandparent Grandchild). Located on the inside of the foot at the base of the bone which makes up the arch of the foot on the same side as the big toe, this point fortifies the spleen, regulates gynecological disorders, and is used with Pc 6 to calm the spirit (in hormonal disorders). Sp 4 has a calming effect on the womb and can safely be used during pregnancy.

Metal: Creation of the Physical Structure That Becomes the Breath of Life

Eastern medicine teaches that there are many ways to improve our bodies and make them fertile. We can eat right, reduce stress, and improve blood flow to the reproductive organs.

But according to Eastern philosophy, we can't force life. Letting go is simply an acknowledgement. There is a lot we can do to control certain aspects of our journey, but we cannot control the outcome. When an infertility patient accepts this truth, she calms the internal fight that keeps her nonreceptive. One of the greatest paradoxes of all times is that when you give up an attachment to results, you are more likely to experience results, according to Eastern medical treatments.

One of the main ways you can improve your ability to release stress is by deep belly breathing. We are conditioned to focus our breathing only on the chest, using the intercostal muscles, which the body perceives as a very stressed way to circulate the breath.

Microcosmic Orbit Breathing Exercise

Most depressed and sick people don't breathe fully. Those who are most alive, vibrant, and fertile do. A full breath triggers the respiratory center in the medulla to activate peptides and endorphins, the initiators of your hormonal system. These peptides are released into the central nervous system and circulate throughout the body. The microcosmic orbit , known in Western medicine as the hypothalamic-pituitary-gonadal axis, activates the respiratory center, circulating its messages of relaxation and receptivity throughout the entire body, most notably the hypothalamic–pituitary–ovarian (HPO) axis, focusing on expanding the lower abdomen, increasing pressure, circulation, and oxygenation to the pelvic organs with every breath. Perform this breathing exercise any chance you have.

As you become experienced, the microcosmic breath should begin to flow as a single movement and will be done effortlessly, without even thinking about it (see **Figure 2**).

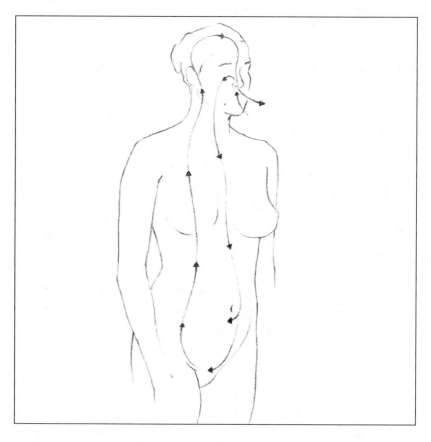

Figure 2: Microcosmic orbit breathing

1. Place tongue on the roof of mouth, behind the front teeth.

2. Inhale through the nose and down the center of the body, through the lungs down the rib cage, letting the diaphragm drop to expand the belly fully.

3. Feel a pool of energy form in your abdomen (the *dan tien*, or source of life).

4. As you are nearing the end of the inhalation, draw the energy down the belly button to the uterus and other abdominal organs and down to the reproductive organs.

5. Perform a very light Kegel exercise by tightening the pelvic floor muscles surrounding the vagina or the perineum. Begin to let your belly fall back in.

6. Release, and as you exhale, visualize the energy rising from the tip of the tailbone and up the spine to the top of the head, down the forehead, and out the nose.

The following are acupressure points that stimulate the relationship between the lungs and the reproductive function.

Lu 7 (Broken Sequence). Found above the wrist crease, about $1\frac{1}{2}$ inches above the prominent bone on the thumb side of the wrist, Lu 7 treats psycho-emotional disorders, regulates the conception vessel, expels wind in the lung, and regulates water balance. This point, along with Ki 6, opens the conception vessel and is often used to "open the upper canopy" at the end of gestation to allow labor to proceed.

Ki 6 (Shining Sea). Located in the depression about one inch below the inner ankle bone, Ki 6 nourishes kidney yin, cools blood, treats infertility and heat disorders, and is helpful for insomnia and amenorrhea. Together with Lu 7, Ki 6 opens the conception vessel.

Fire: The Spirit of Existence, Located in the Heart and Brain Chemistry

Fire energies govern the spirit of life itself, represented by the heart. Chinese medicine focuses on the relationship between the heart and womb as crucial to allowing implantation. The penetrating meridian carries the messages from the heart to the uterus. If this meridian is closed, even the most robust blastocyst will be unable to find a home.

Blood Flow

Traditional Chinese medicine pays quite a bit of attention to the quality of the menstrual flow as one of the main manifestations of menstrual and reproductive health. Uterine linings are considered at least as important as egg quality in Chinese medicine. The attention the body pays to the uterus is directly related to the attention the body pays to the ovary. Chinese medicine considers them a unit, affected also by the messages they receive from the brain chemistry, blood, and hormones. The uterus is an incredibly complex organ whose inner lining is responsible for expressing glandular secretions, proteins, and chemical messages to communicate with the embryo in order for implantation to occur. The honorable term for uterus in Chinese medicine translates to "palace of the child."

Your period should come on every 26 to 32 days. It is normal to experience slight premenstrual tension as progesterone levels drop and the body's energies are directed inward to induce liquefaction of the uterine lining and initiate menstrual flow.

The normal period should last from 3 to 7 days. During this flow period, the normal quantity is expected to be from 50 to 100 milliliters. Lesser flow than 50 milliliters indicates deficiency; more than 100 indicates excess. Here is a rule of thumb to estimate menstrual flow using a regular tampon or pad:

TAMPON	PAD
$\frac{1}{3}$ full = 1 milliliter	$\frac{1}{3}$ full = 1 milliliter
$\frac{1}{2}$ full = 5 milliliter	$\frac{1}{2}$ full = 10 milliliter
full = 10 milliliter	full = 20 milliliter

The color is expected to be fresh to dark red, sometimes with a little bit of brown at the end as the blood flow tapers and oxidizes. If the color is largely brown or black, it indicates the menstrual blood is not able to be released properly; as such, the lining may have difficulty regenerating. Bright red, thin blood that flows rapidly like a fresh cut indicates the lining isn't being properly liquefied along with the blood.

Blood that is too thin and watery also indicates a deficiency in the underlying reproductive energies. If it is thick, clumpy, stringy, or clotty, it indicates an excess condition where the flow is compromised. It should be thicker than a fresh cut, but not so thick it sits on the pad.

Sharp pain is not normal, nor is heavy cramping. A light ache in the center of the pelvis is considered normal, as the contractile function of the uterus is involved in releasing the blood.

For pain relief, use a warm castor oil pack and light massage over the uterus just prior to and during menstruation.

If the consistency is too thick or the color too dark, try supplementing with OPC (oligomeric proanthocyanidins), 125 milligrams per day, and deep sea fish oil, 2000 milligrams per day.

Herbs that help build the uterine lining include the Chinese herb leonurus as well as red raspberry leaf tea and red clover tea.

Acupressure points which address the heart's contribution to the reproductive function include:

Pc 6 (Inner Pass) and Sp 4 (Grandparent Grandchild) (see page 207). These open the penetrating meridian.

Ht 7 (Spirit Gate). Located on the inner wrist crease, toward the base of the hand on the side of the little finger, the Spirit Gate calms the mind and regulates the heart. It is useful in addressing symptoms of heart palpitations, anxiety, agitation, nightmares, depression, mania, insomnia, and restless sleep.

Yintang (Hall of Impression). Located between the eyebrows, yintang is the closest point to the pituitary gland and thus regulates its function. The Hall of Impression calms the mind, allays anxiety and agitation, and resolves frontal headaches. It is often used around the time of implantation and during assisted reproductive techniques.

Performing the exercises described above that enhance blood flow to the uterus and ovaries is also extremely helpful.

Relaxation, Appreciation, and Gratitude

The spirit, governed by the heart and the fire element, reaches its highest potential through the state of relaxation, appreciation, and gratitude, Randine says. Meditation can help open you up to deeper aspects of life. Here is a meditation we like to use on retreat, using soft music and a relaxed position.

Inner Love Meditation

So, here you are, desiring the greatest miracle of all human beings: motherhood. And you may fear it may be denied you. Yet is that really true?

You see, you already embody the essence of motherhood whether or not you have carried a child inside your body, whether or not you have been in the role of somebody's mother. Motherhood comes from within. Check your hands. Feel them from the inside. Are these hands that know how to caress another in need? Do they know to wipe a tear off a cheek? Can they grasp the hand of another and let it know that it is not alone in this life? You have the hands of a mother. Bring your awareness to your arms. Can your strong arms hug the body of one that is not as sturdy as yours is right now? You have the arms of a mother.

Check inside your eyelids. Have your eyes held the sight of love? Have they desired to pass it on? Have they seen another in need and felt the tug to heal them? Your eyes know. They have seen. You have the eyes of a mother.

Check your mouth. Has it kissed? Has it uttered gentle words to make another feel better? Your lips know how to mother.

Bring your awareness to your lap. Is this the lap that patiently waits to fold into an embrace, to allow your gifts of strength, comfort, and nurturing to hold another, accept another, rock and cuddle another, bear another's difficulty, and then let them get up and go on, better for their encounter with you? First, can this lap bear your own burden and release it? You have the lap of a mother.

Check in the depth of your heart. Does it know how to love beyond any love that you may have been able to receive? Does it know how to break open for another? Does it yearn to know that another tender life is just as, even more precious than, its own? Then your heart knows how to mother.

You wear the body of the mother. You carry the heart of the mother. Those are the two most important elements of motherhood. Start to use them now. Give them practice. We know that which we pay attention to grows stronger. Practice them without waiting for the object of your desire. Feel only the energy of your desire, which yearns to love. Practice loving.

No individual soul will choose you based upon your special personality, your unique talents or life situation. Life comes through if certain conditions have been met, and if there is an opening. Practice living life. Rehearse your readiness so that the essence of motherhood can shine through you.

Use your hands to caress. Use your arms to embrace. Use your lips to utter words of tenderness. And let your heart use you. According to Eastern traditions, this is the essence of motherhood.

CHAPTER SIXTEEN

The Benefits
of Genetic Testing

LISA NASH HAS said that she and her husband, Jack, were "twice blessed" by a type of genetic testing offered by our clinic.

"Without this technique, it could have been just Jack and me looking at pictures on the wall instead of raising a family," she said.

The process Lisa referred to is *preimplantation genetic diagnosis* (PGD), an extremely useful and relatively new tool for those seeking to have a child. Do not allow the dry scientific name to fool you. PGD is an incredible advancement that saves lives and spares families great anguish. This wonderful yet controversial tool played a pivotal role in what is probably the most compelling and dramatic case we've ever had—one that became news around the world: Lisa and Jack Nash's genetic diagnosis helped them to have two children—*and* to save the life of one of them.

PGD has become a hot topic in our field and one of the most searched and discussed items on the Internet. The science of PGD begins with this simple fact: Birth defects occur in nearly 5 percent of pregnancies. These defects range from minor physical abnormalities to serious genetic disorders and mental retardation. Some couples, as Lisa and Jack Nash did, have a greater than average risk for creating a child with a serious birth defect. Our clinic helped pioneer the use of genetic diagnosis in combination with in vitro fertilization to reduce the risk for those couples.

PGD allows for the detection of disease-causing mutations and chromosomal abnormalities in embryos prior to conception. Our clinic performed one of the world's first PGD trials, and we have found it to be a vital tool for many of our patients, especially for older women seeking to become pregnant, and for those with known chromosomal abnormalities, gene disorders, and a history of miscarriages.

We knew PGD was an important tool, but the true significance became apparent when we met a young lady, about 6 years of age, named Molly Nash. She was born on July 4, 1994, at Rose Medical Center in Denver. Molly was missing both thumbs. Her right arm was 30 percent shorter than her left. These were recognized as symptoms of Fanconi anemia, a blood disorder characterized by a deficiency of red blood cells, white blood cells, and platelets.

Those born with Fanconi anemia have increased risk for cancer and congenital birth defects. The disease is often associated with cardiac, kidney, and limb abnormalities. Short stature is common in children and adults with Fanconi anemia. They often bleed and bruise easily and have hormonal and fertility problems. Many with this disorder do not survive beyond young adulthood as a result of leukemia or other cancers that cause bone marrow failure. Individuals with Fanconi anemia may pursue bone marrow transplantation, but so far there has been no consistently effective treatment.

Molly had Fanconi anemia type C. Although there are five subtypes of Fanconi anemia, it is only type C that occurs with increased frequency among individuals with Ashkenazi Jewish ancestry. Molly's mother, Lisa, and her father, Jack, both descended from Ashkenazi Jews. It is estimated that approximately one in 89 Ashkenazi Jews is a carrier for Fanconi anemia type C. Parents of an affected child have a 25 percent chance in each future pregnancy to have another child with Fanconi anemia because they are both carriers of the disease.

Molly was facing progressive bone marrow failure unless she was given radiation to kill the diseased cells and then a bone marrow transplant to replace them with healthy cells from a donor. It is a risky procedure, particularly for a child. At the time of Molly's birth, the success rate of a bone marrow transplant from an unrelated donor was 18 percent. But the success rate for transplants from a brother or sister was as high as 65 percent.

Molly was Jack and Lisa's first child, and she had no siblings. That's where our clinic and its ability to perform preimplantation genetic testing entered Molly's treatment program, which would mark the first time in history that medicine combined the sciences of in vitro fertilization, stem cells, and genetic testing. Molly needed the perfect bone marrow donor, which meant a healthy sibling with a tissue match.

PGD was then new and controversial. Yet we thought it would greatly increase the odds that Molly's parents would have another child who would be both healthy and a suitable bone marrow donor for her.

PGD involves testing multiple embryos created by in vitro fertilization. We tested a single cell from each embryo to see if it possessed the genetic mutations that cause Fanconi anemia. Those embryos with the mutations were counted out while the healthy embryos were then tested to see if the tissue type was a match for Molly.

Unfortunately, Jack and Lisa endured four costly but unsuccessful IVF attempts at another clinic before they came to us. Even worse, Molly's health was rapidly declining because of leukemia. Her doctors concluded at one point that time was running out and that Molly could not be saved

"How do you explain to a 5-year-old she's going to die?" her mother asked.

Lisa and Jack came to our clinic as their last hope because we had developed a process for stabilizing an embryo—growing it longer in the Petri dish and giving it a much better chance of implanting. After coming to us, Lisa went through her fifth in vitro in 1 year. This time she produced 24 eggs, almost 3 times as many as she had previously. Half of the embryos were free of the Fanconi anemia mutations. Only one had no traces of Fanconi anemia and was a bone marrow match.

We transferred that single embryo to Lisa's womb on December 15, 1999.

On Christmas Eve, a very weak Molly was undergoing a blood transfusion when my office called her mother to tell her she was pregnant.

It was not an easy pregnancy. Molly's health declined badly in the months that followed. Her parents and doctors weren't always sure the little girl would live long enough to receive her sibling's healthy bone marrow.

On August 29, 2000, Lisa Nash gave birth to a beautiful and healthy baby boy. She named him Adam. Blood from Adam's umbilical cord was harvested and once Molly's diseased bone marrow was destroyed by chemotherapy and radiation, the bone marrow transplant was done. The final part of that life-saving process took all of 25 minutes.

Still, the fight was not over for Molly. She underwent a tortuous recovery. But she survived. She still faces many health challenges because of her genetic condition. We are hopeful, though, that one day, her parents may allow a grown-up Molly and her brother Adam to read the headlines from newspapers around the world that said: "Test-Tube Baby Born to Save His Sister."

Genetics 101

Chromosomes are the structures that contain our genes, which are the blue-prints for our body. Each chromosome looks like a stick and contains 1,000 or more genes. Genes are like the lines of a bar code along the stick (chromo-some). There are 23 pairs of chromosomes, for a total of 46 chromosomes, in each cell of the human body; 23 chromosomes come from the mother's egg and 23 chromosomes come from the father's sperm. The chromosomes are numbered 1 through 22 by size; the twenty-third pair is composed of two X chromosomes (in females) or one X chromosome and one Y chromosome (in males) (see Figure 1).

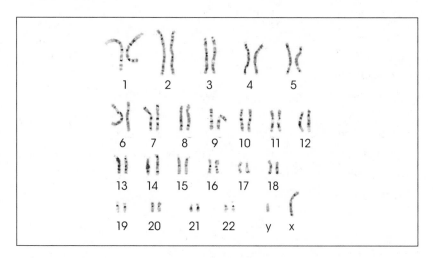

Figure 1: Chromosome pairings

Genetically abnormal embryos may have the wrong number of chromosomes (*aneuploidy;* see also page 223). This is by far the most common genetic problem occurring in embryos. Less commonly, one gene (one line on the bar code) may be abnormal, causing a gene change (mutation) in one of the 25,000 genes that reside in the 23 pairs of chromosomes. Once a genetic abnormality has been identified using PGD, specific PGD techniques are employed to determine which embryos are affected and which embryos are unaffected and available for transfer.

PGD: A Reproductive Option

Mandy Katz-Jaffe, who is director of genetics at our clinic, once worked with babies and children who were born with genetic disorders. The suffering she saw inspired her to work as a reproductive geneticist. "Now, instead of being reactive, I can be proactive," she says. "PGD is an option. It gives women a choice that they did not have before, and that alone is a major advance."

PGD allows us to go into the laboratory and examine developing embryos for disorders even before a patient becomes pregnant. PGD was first developed in the early 1990s to screen embryos for X-linked diseases, such as muscular dystrophy and Klinefelter's Syndrome, which are caused by mutations on an X chromosome.

The technology has expanded to detect countless other genetic disorders and chromosome abnormalities, such as cystic fibrosis, Tay-Sachs disease, Down syndrome, and muscular dystrophy. We can now even screen all 23 pairs of human chromosomes on a single cell. The aim of PGD is to reduce the likelihood of implantation failure, miscarriage, and birth defects by only transferring embryos which are either not affected with a genetic disorder or which have the correct number of chromosomes. PGD is currently the only method available to determine an embryo's genetic status prior to pregnancy.

The PGD Process

Of all of the reproductive options available, PGD is the *only* technique that can be performed before pregnancy. PGD is used to obtain genetic information from the oocyte (egg), day 3 embryo (cleavage stage), or day 5 embryo

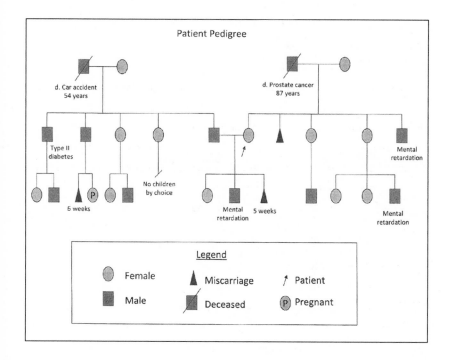

Figure 2: Patient pedigree

(blastocyst), thereby providing an alternative reproductive option for many patients.

The first step, a consultation with a genetic counselor, includes a review of family medical history and construction of a pedigree or family tree (see Figure 2). It is important to note instances of such things as infertility, miscarriage, childhood or infant deaths, and congenital malformations or birth defects in close relatives. A list of any hereditary diseases in either partner's family also is compiled. All of this information helps us look for diseases or syndromes, both hereditary and acquired. The genetic counselor is then able to assess whether there is a risk of having a child with an inherited disorder.

If both partners are identified as carriers for a specific disorder, their chance of having an affected child is 25 percent. The diagnostic information provided by genetic carrier diagnosis allows couples to make better-informed reproductive choices.

PGD for Single-Gene Disorders

One form of PGD is a genetic test offered to couples with a family history of a single gene disorder. Five of the most common disorders for which PGD is used are cystic fibrosis, beta-thalassemia, myotonic dystrophy, Huntington's disease, and fragile X syndrome. PGD is more than 90 percent effective at detecting embryos containing the mutation that will lead to the genetic disorder. This allows couples to begin a pregnancy with an embryo that is not affected by the disease that the parents carry. It also means they don't have to make a decision to therapeutically abort an affected pregnancy. PGD for single gene disorders has been performed for more than 200 different disorders, both with dominant and recessive forms of inheritance.

Biopsy from an Egg

The egg divides its chromosomes in half just before ovulation by ejecting 23 chromosomes out of the egg in a structure called the *polar body*. This polar body can by analyzed without removing a cell from the embryo, thus it is less invasive. This test tells us if the egg is genetically normal and therefore can lead to a normal embryo. Polar body biopsy PGD analyzes the first and second polar bodies (see Figure 3). These structures are discarded by the oocyte during egg maturation and fertilization. The genetic information of both discarded polar

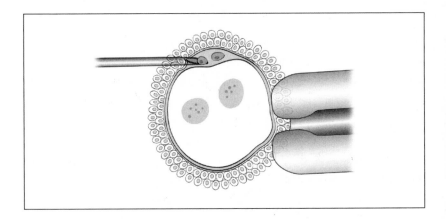

Figure 3: Polar body biopsy

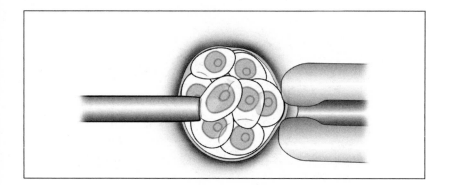

Figure 4: Embryo biopsy

bodies is complementary to the chromosomes remaining inside the oocyte. Polar body PGD is most commonly used in situations where few eggs are collected following ovarian stimulation.

Because polar body PGD does not involve biopsy of the embryo itself, it is valuable for individuals with moral or religious conflicts regarding traditional PGD or for those living in countries with embryo protection laws. The main disadvantage of polar body PGD is that it provides information only about the maternal genetic contribution to the embryo.

Biopsy from a Day 3 Embryo

This most common biopsy for PGD is performed at the cleavage stage or day 3 of embryonic development, when the embryo contains six to eight cells (see Figure 4). On the morning of day 3, one embryo cell is biopsied from the embryo for genetic analysis. In contrast to polar body PGD, this method provides information about both the father's and mother's genetic contributions to the embryo.

Biopsy from a Day 5 Embryo

Blastocyst PGD is performed approximately 5 days after fertilization, when the embryo has differentiated into two cell lines, the *inner cell mass* (ICM) and the trophectoderm (see Figure 5). The ICM will develop into the fetus, and the

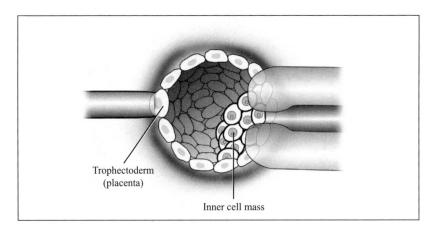

Trophectoderm
(placenta)

Inner cell mass

Figure 5: Blastocyst or trophectoderm biopsy

trophectoderm cells will become the placenta if a clinical pregnancy is established. Cells from the trophectoderm (placenta) are removed without touching
the baby itself (inner cell mass). Typically, biopsied blastocysts are cryopreserved during the time of genetic analysis.

PGD for Chromosomal Abnormalities

Structural chromosomal abnormalities arise when breaks occur in the chromosomes, causing segments to be lost, rotated, or even inserted into neighboring
chromosomes (see Figure 6). An individual with a structural chromosomal
abnormality is often completely normal because he or she has the correct
amount of chromosomal material; it is just rearranged. However, if patients are
carriers for structural chromosomal abnormalities, they have significantly
higher chances of producing eggs or sperm with the incorrect number of chromosomes. This will result in embryos that also have chromosomal errors.

A blood test called a chromosome analysis or *karyotype* can determine which
patients have these structural abnormalities. For such couples, the use of PGD
as a tool for selecting embryos prior to transfer can help to ensure the normal
number of chromosomes in their offspring.

Numerical chromosomal abnormalities, or aneuploidy, are caused during
cell division when the chromosomes do not separate correctly, resulting in too

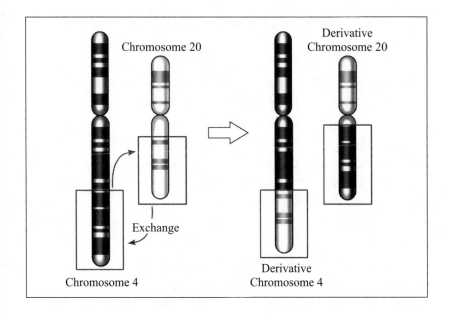

Figure 6: Creation of a balanced chromosomal translocation

many or too few chromosomes in the resulting cells. When aneuploidy occurs during cell division and the formation of the egg or sperm, the resulting embryo will also have the incorrect number of chromosomes.

Chromosome abnormalities have a major impact on embryo viability and are one of the principal causes of failed IVF attempts. Unfortunately, aneuploidy increases with maternal age. In women between the ages of 37 and 40 years, aneuploidy can occur in 50 to 60 percent of eggs, and this increases to 70 percent for women over 40 years of age. The increase in egg aneuploidy seen with advancing maternal age may be associated with the age-related decline in IVF success rates. The lethality of chromosome aneuploidy is also evident in the fact that the majority (approximately 70 percent) of first-trimester miscarriages have an abnormal number of chromosomes. Simply looking at the appearance of the embryo cannot detect chromosome abnormalities. Therefore, it would be reasonable to screen embryos for aneuploidy to identify and transfer only those with the correct chromosome constitution. This should lead to increased pregnancy rates and decreased risks of miscarriage. For these reasons, PGD was developed to screen for chromosome abnormalities and over the past decade has gained popularity in ART procedures.

PGD is recommended to screen for chromosomal abnormalities in cases where the mother is 35 or older, or has had three or more miscarriages, or has had three or more failed IVF cycles or other implantation failure.

Advanced maternal age is a major risk factor for oocyte chromosomal aneuploidy. One of the most common disorders is Down syndrome, which is caused by the presence of an extra chromosome 21. (Its alternative name is *trisomy 21*.) Errors in other chromosomes often lead to embryos that don't implant or that cause early miscarriage. PGD for chromosome aneuploidy aims to prevent these situations in a pregnancy by selecting only normal embryos for transfer.

Recurrent miscarriage is defined as three or more consecutive miscarriages of fetuses between 6 and 20 weeks' gestation. These patients are estimated to include 0.3 to 2 percent of the population. Most of these miscarriages are a result of advanced maternal age, with a high proportion resulting from chromosome aneuploidy. PGD can be used to identify normal embryos and avoid continued miscarriages.

Recurrent IVF failure is defined as three or more failed IVF attempts or implantation failure after the total replacement of more than 10 embryos. The most commonly considered causes of recurrent implantation failure are endometrial abnormalities, advanced reproductive age, and presence of endometrial polyps. Though the potential causes of recurrent IVF failure are diverse, a correlation exists between a higher frequency of chromosomal abnormalities and failed IVF attempts.

PGD Technologies for Aneuploidy Screening

Fluorescent in situ hybridization (FISH) has historically been the chosen procedure of PGD for aneuploidy screening. This technique involves the use of specific fluorescent DNA probes (dots) that stick to the chromosomes and allow them to be counted. Two signals of a particular color indicate that the correct quantity (two copies) of the tested chromosome is present. If an abnormal signal pattern is visualized (that is, one or three signals), the embryo cell is determined to be aneuploid (having the wrong number of chromosomes).

Although initial studies were promising, PGD for aneuploidy screening involving day 3 embryo biopsies and FISH has generated great debate in the past few years regarding the degree to which the procedure improves IVF outcome. Recent studies have failed to show any clinical improvements in IVF outcome. This method only examines between 5 and 9 chromosomes, yet human embryos have 23 pairs of chromosomes. The accuracy of day 3 biopsies with FISH is therefore a problem.

Nevertheless, the concept of PGD for chromosome aneuploidy is not only extremely valuable in that *euploid* embryos (those with the correct number of chromosomes) can be identified and transferred to establish a pregnancy, but also provides patients with diagnostic information regarding their IVF embryos. For example, if no normal embryos are found in one cycle of IVF, the chances of having all abnormal embryos in a subsequent cycle are significantly increased. In this situation, egg donation may be recommended.

Comprehensive Chromosome Screening

Our clinic has been conducting a well-controlled prospective trial using a new method of comprehensive chromosomal screening (CCS). CCS uses two new molecular techniques, *comparative genomic hybridization* (CGH) and *microarray* (MA) technology to screen the entire chromosome complement, all 23 pairs of chromosomes.

CGH (comparative genomic hybridization) and microarray technology are different technologies but appear to be equally effective in testing for all 23 chromosomes.

Our novel CCS strategy involves biopsy of trophectoderm (precursor placental) cells from the embryo at the blastocyst stage (day 5 or 6 of embryonic development). The blastocysts biopsied for PGD need to be cryopreserved (frozen) while genetic analysis takes place to keep them in the best state for transfer. The best IVF success rates are observed using a day 5 embryo.

Our results to date indicate striking improvements in individual embryo implantation rates suggesting that the clinical potential of PGD for chromosome aneuploidy may have been reached with this novel CCS strategy.

We compared patients who underwent day 5 embryo transfers without CCS to our CCS patients. Embryos chosen for transfer in the control group were selected on the basis of traditional appearance (morphological analysis), while those from the CCS study were selected on the basis of chromosome testing. We compared 114 transfers of day 5 CCS embryos to 113 control cycles occurring in the same clinic during the same time period. The control cycles had the same clinical parameters: maternal age, day 3 FSH level, number of oocytes retrieved, fertilization rate, number of blastocysts produced, and number of previous unsuccessful IVF attempts. The probability of one individual blastocyst implanting and forming a pregnancy after transfer was significantly increased in the study group: 65 percent with CCS, compared to 44 percent without screening.

On the basis of this data, we suggest that this CCS strategy, involving blastocyst biopsy, comprehensive chromosome screening, and vitrification with a frozen embryo transfer, has the potential to improve clinical outcome for infertility patients, with increased implantation and single embryo transfer pregnancy rates, as well as reducing miscarriage rates.

Our patient Tracey offered her perspective on the value of PGD in her case:

In 1991, at the age of 20, I was diagnosed with an unknown fertility issue while serving as a Navy Corpsman. Because I was active duty military, I was able to get a wide range of tests and treatments, none of which, unfortunately, led to a successful pregnancy. During my time in the Navy, we tried treatments including ovarian drilling and artificial insemination, but everything failed, and my Navy doctors told me IVF was my only hope.

I got out of the Navy in 2000 and moved to Colorado to be with my husband, Aaron. I was referred to a doctor now working with Dr. Schoolcraft's clinic. Once she'd read the massive medical history of my fight for fertility, she decided to start at ground zero with blood work and sperm samples. We again tried artificial insemination a couple of times without success.

In 2001, we tried another IVF cycle with another doctor who was in the network covered by my insurance. It was unsuccessful and ended in a hyperstimulation. At this time, we decided to cover the cost the best we could and go back to the doctor at Colorado Center for Reproductive Medicine (CCRM). After another round of tests showed everything to be normal, she suggested genetic diagnosis. We agreed because we were desperate for an explanation.

The genetic diagnosis found that my husband had no issues, but I had a chromosome rearrangement that would make it very difficult to conceive. This was devastating news, but after all of the heartache we had already been through, we decided to continue and hope for the best.

Our first round of IVF with genetic screening went forward, and we retrieved four oocytes. Testing showed that only one was suitable for transfer, which we did. This attempt was also, sadly, unsuccessful. We decided to give my body, and our weary spirits, a rest.

In 2003, we decided that we were ready to try again. Then, my husband, who is a US Marine Reservist, was informed that he was being sent to Iraq. We were determined to continue our efforts, so we froze Aaron's sperm before he left. I then began round two, only this time without him there to support me. Still, the day of retrieval was fantastic! We had numerous oocytes, several of which were fertilized through ICSI and sent off for PGD.

PGD results came back, and four or five were suitable genetically and of good quality. While this may not seem like many to most people, it was a treasure trove for us. The day of transfer came, with my husband still in Iraq and me sick as a dog. There were suggestions that I should wait until I felt better, but I had waited so long already I wanted to get it done. Two embryos were transferred that day and they both grew well, initially. We lost one of them in the second trimester, with my husband still deployed.

Finally, on December 17, 2004, our beautiful baby boy, Rhys, was born. Unfortunately, he has the same chromosome rearrangement as I do, which means that he, too, may face challenges when he wants to become a parent.

About 2 years later, Aaron, who had returned safely from Iraq, and I decided that we were ready to attempt the whole process again.

The doctors at CCRM transferred the last two of my frozen embryos. This round went much more smoothly, and I became pregnant. This time only one of the embryos implanted, but on March 6, 2007, our second beautiful baby boy, Owyn, was born, and he has normal chromosomes.

My husband and I highly recommend getting genetic diagnosis done early on versus waiting as long as we did. Knowing whether or not you have a genetic issue can save time, money, and heartbreak. The testing helped us understand our challenges and gave us peace of mind so we could do what we had to do to have a family.

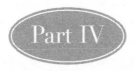

Part IV

Preserving Mind
and Spirit

CHAPTER SEVENTEEN

The Emotional Challenges of Infertility

CHAD AND SHEILA are normally warm and gracious people who wanted a baby so badly that they nearly drove themselves and everyone around them insane. This easy-going, spiritual couple was transformed into a neurotic, controlling, and fire-breathing pair. And that was on their good days. Everything they did, every minute of every day, was focused on getting pregnant and having a baby.

"I swear that if I read on the Internet that eating a whole pineapple raw would help fertility, I'd eat a pineapple every day of the week," Sheila recalled.

It was not funny at the time, but like many couples overwhelmed emotionally by their desire to conceive, once they were able to have a child they looked back and laughed at themselves.

Their case of the "infertility crazies" was not an isolated one, by any means. One of our patients was transformed from a cautious, law-abiding citizen into a serial speeder during her emotion-packed fight to overcome infertility. Another refers to herself as a former "bed rest Nazi" because she kept commanding her gestational surrogate to follow the medical protocol calling for bed rest.

Still other patients say that they invented reasons to sever long-term friendships because they couldn't bear to see other women basking in their pregnancies or bonding with their children. Many have confided that they became virtual hermits during their infertility battles because seeing their friends either pregnant or with children was a constant reminder of what they wanted so desperately and seemingly couldn't obtain. Couples with children are "in the club," whereas couples trying to conceive want nothing more than to be members of what, to them, seems like a difficult club to join.

Few people are prepared for the emotional and psychological toll of infertility, which affects every aspect of our patients' lives. Relationships, finances, careers, religious beliefs, recreational pursuits—all are in some way disrupted and challenged when dealing with infertility. Patients seek the best medical treatment they can afford to deal with the physical issues of infertility, but too often they neglect their psychological and emotional health during this intensely stressful and draining experience.

By balancing mind and body, you can create a sense of calm—essentially making it easier to continue pursuing your dreams of a family. If your mind is calm and your body is healthy, you are better prepared to withstand the trials and tribulations infertility treatments can often bring. The mind-body approach we recommend at the clinic incorporates yoga, meditation, nutrition, massage, acupuncture, and other holistic methods, as well as cognitive-behavioral counseling, which can be done individually or in a group. Our approach focuses on the interactions of the mind, body, and behavior and on the ways in which emotional, mental, behavioral, and spiritual factors affect health.

A Major Event

The men and women who come to us to find solutions to infertility often feel overwhelmed and even panicked. One patient said, "I feel like I'm drowning. I am struggling to stay afloat. Please throw me a life preserver."

In 1998, the Supreme Court ruled that trying to have a child is a "major life activity" covered under the Americans with Disabilities Act. For anyone who has been trying to conceive for more than a year, this was not news. Most of our patients will agree that the challenges of infertility can also constitute a major life crisis.

We tell our patients that for the infertile couple there are four stages of trying to conceive:

1. Trying to conceive naturally

2. Diagnosis of infertility

3. Infertility treatment

4. Resolution of infertility

Each stage has its own level of stress. No one stage is harder to cope with than another. All of these stages involve a sense of loss, and you may experience grief, consciously or unconsciously. Studies have found that men and women dealing with infertility can experience chronic stress on the same level as patients dealing with deadly diseases. Some of the emotions they might experience are:

Depression	Helplessness	Anxiety
Sadness	Anger	Resentfulness
Loneliness	Jealousy	Pessimism
Guilt	Shame	Preoccupation with fertility
Fear	Isolation	Loss of control
Frustration		

We have no doubt that infertility triggers stress. It also may be true, unfortunately, that stress could possibly have an impact on your ability to conceive. There have been published studies offering evidence in varying degree that stress itself may influence the success of fertility treatments. Still, this has been the subject of considerable debate in the medical community.

Let's walk through the stages mentioned earlier and consider some approaches to managing the stress at each stage.

Stage One:
Trying to Conceive Naturally

When a couple decides they are ready for a baby, they typically want to get the pregnancy started *yesterday*. Couples often assume that they will conceive within the first few months. This can lead to feelings of disappointment should a pregnancy not occur quickly. As time passes, concern, fear, and anxiety may begin to replace the initial hope and excitement. After a few months, many couples begin to wonder if something is wrong. A sense of loss may begin to creep over you at this point, bringing feelings of insecurity, disappointment, and a growing fear that you may not be able to have children.

During this time, friends and family may begin to notice that you aren't acting like yourself. Some may express sympathy and understanding. You may choose to confide in them, or you may not. We find that some men and women prefer to keep their concerns about infertility private. Some may feel embarrassed to reveal their concerns.

If you choose to share your feelings about your efforts to have a child, be aware that family and friends may say things that they believe to be helpful or supportive, but they may not understand. Patients frequently say that friends will tell them, "Don't worry, just relax and it will happen." This can trigger anger, frustration, feelings of isolation, and the sense that no one "gets it." It helps to remember that even those who have good intentions and want to support you may come across as rude and hurtful because they don't fully understand or they simply may not know how to be more supportive. Talking to a support group or infertility counselor can help you feel that others understand.

For example, a well-intentioned mother-in-law may tell you, "Oh, just give it time." Or a friend may tell you a story of another couple who began the adoption process and suddenly conceived. They are trying to give you hope, but patients often say it is hard for them to hear such comments when they are struggling to get pregnant. You may find it helpful to explain to friends and family a bit about infertility as well as how they best support you. If you share your needs with others, they are more likely to be able to meet them.

Many people in this stage and beyond find themselves becoming acutely aware of pregnant women, babies, and all things associated with pregnancy. It's normal to feel this way, but a simple trip to the mall may become difficult emotionally as you notice all of the pregnant women waddling through the stores or mothers with what may seem like their multitudes of children.

You may find yourself feeling that life isn't fair when you see other new mothers and their children. You are in a heightened sense of awareness when it comes to parenthood and this can trigger stress. To make it even more challenging, while you are feeling more stressed than ever, your well-meaning friends, family, and others are constantly telling you to "just relax." Right? So, you really aren't going crazy. We hear this from patients all the time.

Stage Two: Diagnosis of Infertility

Typically, patients come to us after trying unsuccessfully to conceive for 6 to 12 months or longer. In our initial conversations, they talk about feeling afraid, sad, hopeful, and eager; in other words, their emotions are all over the map. Men and women may experience entirely different emotions. Often couples fall into the blame game at this point. One may blame the other, but often, each of them feels responsible in some way. We advise our patients to avoid that trap. Infertility is a medical challenge, and we work with them to find a solution. There is no reason to blame either partner. You and your partner are in this together, trying to achieve a common goal. And your clinic team is there to help you.

Keep in mind that you will get through this, and hopefully your relationship will be even stronger. You and your partner may have very different thoughts and feelings about infertility, and you may choose to cope with it very differently. An experienced counselor specializing in infertility can help the two of you find a common ground in your mission to start a family.

Following the diagnosis of infertility, a couple may be forced to make a decision. You may end up choosing to pursue fertility treatments such as *intrauterine inseminations* (IUI, or artificial inseminations), in vitro fertilization, donor egg or donor sperm, to adopt a child, or not to have children after all. The decision-making period can be very stressful, too. There are often many factors of pregnancy and parenthood to consider, such as feelings about the time and cost involved and religious beliefs, just to name a few.

Often, couples look for guidance: "I just wish someone would tell me what to do." Yet this is such a personal matter, and such a life-changing decision, that you really have to make this choice together. It is also true that it's rare for both partners to feel exactly the same way about all the options you face. It is important to respect each other's opinions, but eventually you will have to come to an agreement on your treatment plan. We encourage couples to explore their values and priorities so they can find a solution together.

The Fertility Crazies

Couples at this point tend to experience "the fertility crazies." This happens when you are no longer thinking or acting like your "old self" because you are stressed out like never before. Does it help to know that feeling a little crazy is pretty normal? We have a counseling team at our clinic for that reason. We also offer acupuncture, massage, yoga, and mild exercise as ways to relieve the stress and to make you feel more in control of your emotions.

Stage Three: Infertility Treatment

While pursuing infertility treatment, it is quite common to experience extreme emotional highs and lows. This is commonly referred to as the infertility roller-coaster. It can be a rough ride. Couples often report excitement and hope at the beginning of a treatment cycle, and disappointment and despair should a pregnancy not occur. Your highs and lows may well seem higher and lower than usual because of the intense stress, coupled with hormonal treatments your doctors may prescribe. This is another reason we have so many patients tell us they feel "out of control" and that their daily lives have become more difficult. Counseling can help you deal with those feelings.

We also hear patients say they feel like a "human pincushion" throughout their infertility treatment. No wonder; treatment often requires frequent blood draws, vaginal ultrasounds, and hormone shots. You will likely feel physically and emotionally drained, so it is important to take care of yourself in both departments. Many patients find it helps to keep a journal of their feelings and experiences. Regular exercise, yoga, soothing music, and trips to the beach or mountains can help ease the stress. We remind our patients often to keep their eyes on the prize—a baby in your buggy.

Additional concerns that may arise during infertility treatments include a feeling that your time is no longer your own; that your quest for fertility is dominating your life. Your doctor may want to see you at very specific times on specific days in order to monitor your cycles. This can conflict with commitments at work or at home.

The frustration can be magnified if you choose not to disclose your situation to your employer or coworkers. Additionally, you may find it difficult to schedule vacations and other trips. Again, we encourage you to keep your eyes on the prize. You are going through this for a very good cause, to build your family. The inconveniences are only temporary, but the rewards can last a lifetime. If you can maintain a sense of balance and fit fertility treatment into your life rather than stopping "life" for fertility treatment, you may feel better.

Now that we've reminded you of the rewards, let's talk about the bills. Financial concerns arise for most people involved in infertility treatments because most health plans don't cover all aspects, if any. Infertility is generally not something that is planned; therefore, most people haven't established an "infertility fund." Treatments are expensive and can put couples in a pinch. We encourage patients to put their financial concerns into perspective. There is no denying that infertility treatments are expensive, but you are spending this money for a great cause. Often, people spend $20,000 for a car without flinching; you shouldn't flinch when it comes to spending money on your *child*. Still, patients should remain within their financial comfort zones.

Stage Four: Resolution of Infertility

Arriving at this stage means one of three things: either a pregnancy has occurred, you have chosen to adopt a child, or you have decided to remain childless. No one option is better than another. As mentioned earlier, it really is an individual decision; no one can make it for you.

Most clinics offer counseling suited to every possible option. One of the things we remind people at this stage is that you will still face challenges down the road. Parenting can be very different for the couple who has experienced infertility. Often, having a baby or adopting a baby after a long fertility journey can trigger additional fears and anxiety. Couples who do start their families after experiencing infertility say they are far more protective of their child than couples who have not had to work so hard to do it.

Women who finally become pregnant after struggling with infertility may have heightened fears about the pregnancy and the baby. If you feel an over-whelming anxiety, please talk to a counselor about your situation. There are proven methods to relieve your stress, and you don't want to let anxiety cause more problems for you.

Deciding not to become a parent is another option. Some find fulfillment being aunts, uncles, or mentors instead of parents. People can lead very fulfill-ing lives without having children of their own. Couples who choose this lifestyle can focus on other aspects of their lives, such as relationships, hobbies, travel, and careers.

Coping with the Stress of Infertility

During each of the stages above, you need to take care of yourself. Take the time for relaxing activities; exercise, socialize, and don't forget to laugh. Some-times patients get so focused on having a child they neglect themselves. But if you are successful in having a child, that little person will need you to be healthy and happy, too.

So, schedule time for personal maintenance. Pencil in "me time" on the cal-endar, whether it is taking a walk, reading a book, or writing in a journal. Find coping mechanisms you enjoy. If you hear inner voices telling you, *I'm not meant to be a parent*, or, *Nothing ever works out for me*, or, *I'm never going to be happy*, a counselor can help you reframe those messages and find more constructive thoughts.

Patients sometimes comment that they feel they need to be positive or fertil-ity treatment will never work. I also hear from patients that being positive is just too much of a stretch. You don't have to put on a smiley face if you aren't in the mood. Optimism is helpful, but not mandatory. We encourage patients to be in the moment. Express whatever emotion you are feeling. Don't feel com-pelled to be upbeat all the time.

Another useful tool is to find a neutral feeling. If thinking positively is too much of a stretch but negative thoughts are dragging you down, a good neutral position might be this thought: "I'm doing everything I can to get pregnant." It is neither positive nor negative and keeps you focused on the present.

Life tends to get out of balance when you are dealing with infertility. Your relationships, your work, and nearly every other aspect of your life is affected.

Some patients tend to isolate themselves; they say friends and family "don't get it." Your work may suffer because of all the doctor appointments. Your relationship with your partner may be strained due to differing perspectives, changes in your sex life, and financial constraints.

People in our care often tell us that they feel their only identity becomes that of a fertility patient. That can be a tough role to play. We see patients lose self-esteem and fall into depression or suffer anxiety and confusion.

Most clinics have fertility counseling teams to help patients find balance in their lives even amid all the demands and stress of their treatment. These counselors strive to help patients find strength by focusing on the positives in their lives and on the ultimate goal of having a child. At our clinic, we provide patients with three basic tools to help them deal with the emotional challenges of infertility:

1. **Compartmentalization.** We ask patients to visualize a wall of shelves with many different shoe boxes. Then we note that you can only wear one pair of shoes at a time, just as you can only focus on one concept at a time. When you are at work, focus on work. When you are with friends, concentrate on shared interests rather than your own infertility fight. We remind patients that they can't always focus on their infertility treatments if they want to maintain a healthy balance in their lives. Compartmentalization may be easier for men than women, but can be very helpful for both partners nonetheless.

2. **Mental vacation.** Even the small things can wear us out if we dwell on them all the time. We demonstrate this by asking patients to hold a bottle of water overhead for a minute, then for five minutes. It's small, so the short period isn't a problem, but the longer you try to hold it up there, the heavier it seems to get. In the same way, holding one thought for too long can become a burden. So, rather than always thinking about infertility, give your mind a break; take mental vacations to relieve the burden. We recommend reading, watching movies, or pursuing some other interest that takes your mind off infertility matters.

3. **Beware of snow balls.** It is very easy for one small thought to "snowball" and grow to a massive size in a very short time. We often have patients whose

negative thoughts "snowball" into nightmarish thoughts, so that the thought "This IVF cycle isn't going well" grows into "I'll never have my own family." We encourage patients to stay focused on step-by-step treatments and on the ultimate goal rather than dwelling on the worst possible scenarios.

The bottom line is you can survive the stress of dealing with infertility. Thousands of our patients have done it. An amazingly high percentage of those who come to us with infertility diagnoses eventually find a path to fertility and a family.

The fertility crazies is not a permanent condition. It's natural to feel some stress, but there are proven ways to ease your mind and lift your spirit, even in the most challenging situations. Your clinic counselors are there to help you, so make use of their talents.

Mars and Venus during the Fertility Fight

When couples come to us for counseling to address the emotional challenges related to infertility, one of the first things we try to explain is that men and women tend to approach infertility from their own distinct "Mars" or "Venus" perspective.

Let's face it: when there is a problem, most men want to fix it. They are not interested in talking about their feelings or analyzing their experiences. Men are conditioned to ignore feelings and focus on action—on finding a solution.

Think about the most sensitive man you know. Even he has difficulty knowing how to verbalize his emotions, doesn't he? Women, on the other hand, are all about expressing their feelings and emotions. When facing a problem, women usually want to share their emotions. Most of all, they want others to understand their feelings.

The differing Mars-Venus perspectives can be magnified when facing a challenge as intense as infertility. We often find that when couples are first told by a doctor that there is a fertility problem, the males tend to take the optimistic approach, while the women are more inclined to express despair and frustration.

Most men hold on to the belief that medical science will find a way to solve the problem until a doctor tells them otherwise. Many women, on the other hand, remain skeptical or unbelieving until a delivery room nurse puts a baby in their arms.

We also find that while going through fertility treatment woman usually are more ready to jump to the next treatment option or to explore the possibility of adoption, while men tend to believe conception will happen if they just keep trying. Again, this may be attributed to his optimism or her tendency to feel more emotionally compelled to have a child to mother. Whichever the case may be, if we peer into the minds of men and women in the early stages of the fertility fight, we often find that men tend to feel "pressured" to keep trying by the women, while women feel "held back" by the men.

Once the initial shock of the infertility diagnosis wears off, women want to keep talking about it, often to the point of obsessing over it. This may be attributable to many things, but the most likely causes are biology and sociology. Biologically speaking, women have a limited number of years when their bodies can conceive and carry a baby successfully. As their biological clocks tick on, women are mindful that they have a limited number of eggs and a limited time to get them fertilized before their quality declines.

Women are the designated baby carriers, so infertility treatments deal primarily with them even if the male has the fertility challenge. Women typically bear most of the emotional burden of infertility, too. For most women, the tender dream of motherhood begins in childhood play and continues to be an important part of her physical and emotional development through her adolescence and into adulthood.

The dream of motherhood also permeates her relationships and social interactions. Women in their child-bearing years tend to bond with each other around their shared desire to get pregnant, then around their pregnancies, their deliveries, and raising their children. So, when a woman is struggling with infertility, she often feels left out of those bonding sessions. It's the same for couples. As friends, family members, and coworkers start their families, the childless couple feels left behind, isolated, and even shunned. Although this may not be intentional on the part of those close to them, the couple dealing with infertility can feel that they've been locked out of the "parents club." After all, it is one thing to choose not to have children, but quite another to be unable to conceive or bear them.

Frustrations and Stresses

We find that as the infertility treatment process unfolds, many men begin to feel frustrated and more and more helpless. They want to find a solution and fix the problem. Patience is not always a virtue they embrace, especially when they are dealing with a distressed female partner. No matter what resources are at hand, no matter how skillful the treating physician and the clinic team may be, men often express anger and frustration that they cannot fix this problem. They want to help their female partners, and when they can't find a quick solution, it stresses them out.

These can be difficult times for a couple. The woman expresses her feelings. The man responds by suggesting solutions. His response to her words—rather than to her feelings—triggers the age-old lament, "You're not listening to me. You just don't get it."

She wants him to feel the intensity of her emotional pain. His instincts are to find a solution instead. Women infertility patients often tell us that they feel their lives are spinning out of control. Women spend countless hours research-ing infertility and treatment options in order to regain control. Sadly, some go to extremes, following unproven "fertility diets" or embracing the latest fertility "miracle cure" peddled on the Internet or in the tabloids.

Men, on the other hand, do not feel like their lives are of control because they are better able to compartmentalize infertility. We find that the male typi-cally defers to the female as she immerses herself in research and becomes the "expert" on infertility and treatment options. The female partner may interpret this to mean that the male is not as involved in the process or not as upset about it. The truth is that he is very likely hurting and does feel the pain; he just handles it differently. We often have to help our female patients understand that the male partner may be undergoing more stress and emotional pain than she realizes.

If considerable amounts of time pass and despite all the expensive tests and treatments, there is still no baby, men often will struggle with how to cope with the disappointment and with the woman's highly charged emotions. Men often express their frustration saying, "I can't say anything right. I can't do anything right."

The woman's view is that he doesn't let her express her emotions, or that he doesn't listen when she tries to. "He won't talk about it. He just shuts down." His view is that "it's all she talks about, day and night. She is obsessed with having a baby. Why?"

He wants this problem solved. He wants his wife back. For women, the stress and intensity of emotions associated with infertility can be overwhelming and very uncomfortable. She needs to vent, and the male partner often feels the heat and bears the brunt of her anger and frustration. Men tend to withdraw in these situations, which, in turn, leads her to conclude that he doesn't care enough or that he isn't really interested in starting a family with her.

Money and Sex Issues

As if gender communication differences were not enough, infertility challenges also stir up the two most notorious relationship demons: money and sex. With infertility challenges, a couple does not get to have a bottle of chardonnay and make a baby the old fashioned way. Instead of enjoying intimacy in the bedroom, they find themselves in the sterile environment of a clinic, talking to medical professionals who ask the most personal of questions and poke and prod their most private parts. Then, they have the audacity to charge for all the expensive tests and treatments. And treatment is often not covered by health insurance.

Financially, the fertility fight can be devastating for couples. For many men, this aspect of infertility is the most stressful. Women may become so emotionally caught up in the desire to have a child that they overlook the financial toll. "You can't put a price tag on your own child," women often say. Between his partner's attitude and the size of the bills, a man can feel backed into a corner. The stress can seem unbearable.

Sexual intimacy also can suffer during the fertility fight. Nearly 50 percent of all couples going through fertility treatment report a decrease in sexual activity, not to mention a sharp decline in sexual satisfaction. This is no surprise, given the fact that sex, which was previously a lighthearted, intimate experience, is now constantly being analyzed, discussed, charted, and reviewed by your medical team.

Spontaneous sex gives way to carefully plotted, planned, scheduled, and chronicled encounters that feel like clinical exercises. When sex becomes choreographed by doctors and nurses bearing thermometers and calendars, the thrill is gone.

For both men and women, this creates a problem, obviously. There is the often unspoken resentment men feel when pressured to perform on demand or to serve as "sperm-producing machines" in the clinic.

Self-Image Issues

Sex can also affect the way a woman feels about her body, especially while she's being treated for infertility. Over the years, we've often heard women share their most private and intimate thoughts on this topic. For many but certainly not all women facing infertility, sex can be a constant reminder that their body has failed to produce a child. This feeling of failure can become pervasive. It can affect not only the way a woman perceives her body but even her perception of herself as a woman.

We've had patients tell our counselors that they feel like "less of a woman" or "incomplete as a woman" because they can't conceive. Women also have shared fears that their male partners might abandon them for a woman who is more fertile. Our response to these fears is to remind our women patients that their partners want to have a child with them, not just any woman.

It's also true that issues of threatened sexuality and masculinity can arise for men dealing with infertility, especially if they are diagnosed with a low sperm count or other fertility challenge.

Sharing Your Situation

In our counseling with patients, we offer tools for coping with the emotional, financial, and mental challenges that come with infertility. We encourage the male and female partners to help each other get through it. But then they also have to deal with questions and pressures from people outside their relationship.

To tell or not to tell? Whom to tell and when? These are common questions men and women ask themselves; however, unlike so many other issues related to infertility, their decisions on whom to tell and when to tell don't seem to be based on gender so much as on their feelings about privacy.

As much as we try to counsel them otherwise, many women feel ashamed when dealing with infertility. Overwhelmed with sadness, guilt, and confusion, some women will shut down their social networks and isolate themselves. As long as the male partner is in agreement, that may work for a couple. Yet when one partner feels the need to talk about infertility with loved ones and the other partner doesn't, more conflict can result.

We encourage couples to work out what they want to do before conflict begins. The man and woman should discuss how much they want to share, with whom they want to share it, and at what point they want to start sharing. In truth, most couples seem to work this out. As time passes, men and women recognize that they can endure only so much alone and that it is helpful to talk to supportive people—be they understanding loved ones, friends, or people in support groups who "get it."

Amazingly, couples do survive infertility in spite of these gender differences. The key is to recognize that when facing a crisis, men and women handle things differently, and as a very wise person once told me, "different is just different." There is not one way or even a best way to handle a crisis. Instead, each person must figure out what they need from their mate, communicate these needs on a regular basis, and take turns "playing nice" with each other.

Melissa and Mark discovered this. They came to counseling because they were stuck in trying to make a decision on whether or not to pursue an IVF cycle. They could not agree, and they were fighting with each other. During their first counseling session, Melissa explained that they had tried three Clomid cycles but none had been successful. She also told us that because their infertility was unexplained, their doctor had recommended that they pursue an IVF cycle.

With tears in her eyes, Melissa said she didn't understand why Mark would not consider doing an IVF cycle. She felt it made sense because the process often gives doctors more information so they can diagnose exactly what is causing the infertility.

Mark said he had several concerns about the IVF cycle, including the cost and the fact that there is no guarantee it would produce a pregnancy. He told Melissa that since they were young, "there's no reason why we shouldn't get pregnant soon. We just need to keep trying. It will happen."

At last report, this couple was attending counseling and trying to see one another's side of the issue. But it is not easy for them, especially because Melissa has many pregnant friends, and she feels she is missing out on their shared experience. After several counseling sessions, both Mark and Melissa said they felt like "wounded warriors" in their quest for fertility. Yet at least they learned to face this battle together. Thankfully, the couple is learning to communicate more effectively with one another, to take breaks from the issue, and to confide in people they trust. Thanks to their support group, they also realize that they are not alone, that there is still hope, and that one day, they will become parents.

CHAPTER EIGHTEEN

Working Well
with Your Fertility Team

WE HAD JAYLYNN covered. We'd done weeks of tests on her and on the woman she'd chosen as her egg donor. Then, all our carefully planned schedules for her treatments were thwarted by a single tattoo.

The woman serving as JayLynn's egg donor had a rose tattooed on her ankle. Tattoos and body piercings may be fashionable, but they carry a high risk of infection. As a result, clinics are required by law to reject egg donors who have had tattoos or body piercings done within a year of a match with recipients. These laws are established to maintain public safety and they can't be circumvented.

News of the delay in her treatment sent JayLynn off the deep end, which was understandable. Unfortunately, she took it out on her nurse and other staff members. She unleashed her frustration with a barrage of verbal abuse that sent everyone within earshot scrambling for cover. Maybe JayLynn needed to vent, but her explosive outburst brought extensive collateral damage.

JayLynn had to do some serious damage control. Even so, the nurse who took the brunt of her anger decided that she could no longer work with JayLynn. Even JayLynn's husband was upset with her for alienating staff members and further delaying their efforts to have a child.

The nurses and other staff members at my clinic do not usually share their personal stories with patients, but many of them first came to our clinic as patients. Several were working in other areas of medicine, such as surgery, emergency room, delivery room, or neonatal care, until they had to deal with infertility themselves. Their personal experiences made them realize the great need for sympathetic medical professionals in this arena.

Even seasoned health care pros are surprised at the intensity of the experience when they begin working with infertility patients. Veterans of those high-stress environments find that infertility patients can be extremely difficult to work with because the emotional strain of the process can make patients volatile.

Helping the Staff Help You

Everyone wants to be treated with respect and without animosity. This chapter offers guidance to help patients interact effectively with doctors, nurses, and other staff members during treatment for fertility. Honest communication is essential. We need to know how you are feeling physically and emotionally so we can treat you effectively. Building an effective working relationship with your treatment team is essential.

Our doctors, nurses, and other infertility staff members want you to be comfortable in communicating with them, so tell them what methods work best for you. We can make adjustments for language barriers, learning styles, and privacy concerns. We can help you overcome frustrations by giving you as much information as you think you can handle. Some patients want in-depth details and medical and scientific explanations. Others say, "Just tell me what to do and when to do it."

Even patients from medical professions have questions about the infertility and treatment options available, so don't feel self-conscious about asking your fertility team for answers. We don't want to overwhelm you with information, yet we want you to feel that you are getting all that you need from us.

Having trust in your caretaker makes the process go infinitely smoother. Our patient Clara was typical in that she had a series of setbacks from miscarriages and failed cycles at other clinics before she came to us. She was very nervous, but she reached out to her nurse and shared her feelings and her fears. Clara said she'd had six previous miscarriages, and she felt alone in her grief. She'd had a bad experience at another clinic, where she felt they didn't support her after a miscarriage. She also said that she could no longer talk about her grief with her husband because he would break down in tears, upset that he couldn't "make it better."

Clara also was having trouble dealing with the fact that her sister was pregnant. "I want to be happy for her, but seeing her just makes me sadder that I can't get pregnant," she said. Clara didn't want to burden her mother with her issues or intrude on the joy of her sister's pregnancy.

This patient was carrying a heavy load. The staff, including the primary nurse, rallied to support her by listening to her and consoling her. Patients should understand that not all clinicians are good with helping people through grief and loss. It's not that they don't care. It's just that dealing with patients' frustration and grief can be difficult for health care providers trained to treat physical illness rather than emotional trauma. Some doctors and nurses may appear unconcerned because they are focused on looking for medical solutions rather than on offering sympathy and understanding.

Clara was very respectful of the fact that her treatment team had many patients to care for. She noted this in her many emails and phone calls. She gave the team time to get back to her. She respected their time by saving up her questions and asking them when her nurse had time to devote to her. Her treatment team appreciated Clara's thoughtful approach, and, as a result, they tried to be just as thoughtful in their dealings with her.

Clara's difficult fertility journey was eased by her good rapport with her nurse, which carried over to other staff members. When it was time for Clara's pregnancy test, the phlebotomist, the surgical nurse, and the genetic counselor all enjoyed helping Clara. This became obvious when the entire team gathered for a phone call to tell Clara the good news, shouting over the speaker, "Congratulations, Clara, you are pregnant!"

Clara's willingness to be open and share her feelings, frustrations, and disappointments in a manner that was not hostile or accusatory helped her develop a supportive rapport with a team that was there to listen and help her through her journey. Patients like Clara generally have a better experience.

Too often, patients unleash their angers, fears, and even jealousy on their nurses, doctors, or other staff. We've had young nurses assailed by overwrought patients who resented their youthful fertility or the fact that they were pregnant.

Some infertility patients go to the other extreme. They see their nurses as the gateway to their goals and try to please them and earn their favor by telling them what they think the nurses want to hear. That doesn't usually work well either.

Treatment and Commitment

Your treatment team understands that most patients need to share their medical histories and their stories with staff. Your clinic should provide you with ample opportunities to do this. Initially, you will meet with a physician who will evaluate your medical history and the best treatment option. You will most likely feel overwhelmed by all the questions asked during this consultation. Think of it as entering information into a computer. The more good information you give it, the better results you get from its computations.

Even with that in mind, you can expect emotional highs and lows as part of the experience. Typically, you will be assigned a primary nurse who will help support you in your journey. The first step will involve setting up a consultation to review the entire process, which can be very daunting. Both partners should view this as an essential meeting. There is far too much information imparted for any one person to absorb. Both of you should attend and take notes so you can compare them later. We've had problems crop up during treatment because patients or their partners did not attend or pay attention during this important meeting.

Our patient Karla came to the consult alone. She explained that her husband, David, was just too busy with his business to get away. "I will just give him the information he needs to know," she said.

We were concerned about this but let it slide, though we regretted it later. The problem is that there is so much information that it is difficult for a spouse to relay it all to the partner. Think of the toughest science course you took in high school. Now imagine taking the entire course in one day!

The nurse consultation typically reviews guidelines including:

○ Dos and don'ts

○ Risks

○ Medication instructions and possible side affects

- Possible pregnancy issues and outcomes

- Genetic testing recommendations

- Workup calendar

- Cryopreservation

- Consents

- Costs

- Review of retrieval and transfer

- Emotional issues to expect throughout the cycle

- Time commitment

As you can see, this is a great deal of information to absorb, let alone to try and relay to someone else.

Karla found out just how difficult it can be. Prior to their consultation, Karla's husband completed his workup. His semen analysis was normal. Then the couple went on to their IVF cycle. David gave his semen sample only to discover his semen analysis count was extremely poor. The embryology team informed David that they found no motile sperm in the sample.

He had to recollect a sample but again there were no motile sperm in the sample. The couple was devastated. They could not understand what went wrong with the sample. They wondered how normal samples could turn so quickly to abnormal samples—and at the most critical time the sample was needed to create embryos.

The physician asked David and Karla whether they had made any lifestyle changes. At first, the couple could not think of anything that might have affected David's sperm count. After further discussion, David mentioned that he was a farmer and that he'd been sitting for prolonged periods in his combine machine harvesting in extremely hot weather. If David had attended the initial session, he would have learned that extreme temperature exposure can have a serious impact on his sperm count.

Because of David's poor semen count, the couple's IVF cycle was canceled. The couple was devastated. Karla had followed the dos and don'ts, but the male partner's dos and don'ts during the IVF cycle did not get passed on to David.

The physicians recommended that David retest 6 months after completing his next harvest on the farm. The goal was to evaluate whether the extreme temperature exposure was the culprit to his poor sperm performance. That turned out to be the case. Measures were taken to make sure David and his reproductive parts did not get overheated. The couple repeated an IVF cycle and, thanks to more mobile sperm from David, they were successful in achieving a twin pregnancy.

There is a method to our madness. We request that the male and female come together for our initial consultations because they both need to process the information we provide.

The Best Policy

Being honest about your medical history and all other information is essential. Do not worry about shocking medical professionals. What feels silly or embarrassing to you is usually old hat to them, and it could be very important in your treatment.

We all understand that you've been asked to share information about a very intimate aspect of your life, and perhaps the most intimate aspect of your relationship. Your treatment team is there to help, not pass judgment. We need to understand your feelings, including your fears.

Your doctors, nurses, and other clinic staff are accustomed to frank and open discussions about sexual intercourse and menstrual cycles. One of our nurses was reminded of the unusual nature of our work when her middle school son, who was taking sex education at the time, came home and informed her that he'd taken a poll and found that no other kid in middle school had "sperm magnets" on his refrigerator.

She explained that the magnets from the office had pictures of embryos, not sperm, on them.

Then her son came up with another zinger: "Why do you have to call people on the phone and tell them to have sex at night?"

Fighting to control her laughter, our nurse mom explained that her job is to help couples have babies and sometimes that meant encouraging them to be together at just the right time.

Her young and observant son seemed satisfied with that explanation, for the time being. So, as this nurse's experience illustrates, we are not easily shocked. Being honest and following instructions helps build trust with your treatment team and helps them build trust in you. We need to know that we can depend on each other as we work toward our shared goal.

Trust is essential because we work so closely with you in this most intimate part of your life. Lack of trust only causes frustration. It slows down the process, and nobody wants that. We want to take you from patient to parent as quickly and smoothly as we can.

The policies and procedures at most reputable fertility clinics are established by their medical teams to make certain that each patient has a complete and comprehensive evaluation prior to attempting pregnancy. These evaluations are designed to protect patients as well as lowering the risks to their potential pregnancies.

Sharon was excited when she called the nurse to inform her that she started her cycle and was ready to *start a calendar*. As you've no doubt already noticed, infertility clinics have their own language. This is a commonly used term in our line of work. When a patient begins preparing for the IVF cycle, a calendar is made showing what will happen each day and when the anticipated retrieval and transfer of embryos will be done. So when a patient is ready to start a calendar, it means she is beginning her IVF cycle.

Sharon was 46 years old, and her heart health was not an obvious concern. But when it came time for her to start her calendar, the nurse informed Sharon that she had not done her required cardiac evaluation. The patient said she had forgotten but would schedule this right away. Sharon was adamant that she wanted to start her calendar prior to getting the cardiac workup results. She blamed her nurse, saying she was never told to complete the cardiac exam.

Information on the cardiac exam is always provided during the initial nurse consultation as well as in patient handouts. The nurse reviewed again that the testing for patients over 45 years old includes a full cardiac evaluation because some of the more common chronic diseases may be present in women over 45. She explained to Sharon that some of the chronic diseases include arthritis, hypertension diabetes, eclampsia, preeclampsia, placental abruption, and even strokes.

Proper evaluation increases the awareness of heart risk factors and other chronic diseases among pregnant women. But Sharon was so focused on getting pregnant that she had put her own health at risk. She became very angry with the nurse for telling her she could not have a calendar.

Sharon begged, pleaded and demanded to start her donor's calendar. She asked her physician and nurse to waive the recommended cardiac test.

"I am completely healthy person, I live a healthy life style, and it is ridiculous to think that I am at any cardiac risk. I have to get pregnant before I turn 47 years old, and it has already taken 3 months to find this donor," she stated.

The physician refused to allow her to skip the cardiac testing. The nurse did give her a calendar, though, as a way to show the patient she trusted her to complete the testing. Sharon and her donor began the costly medication regime.

Three days before the scheduled egg retrieval, Sharon had her EKG and cardiac stress test. The results showed that she had significant cardiac blockage. The cardiologist explained the stress of pregnancy could have been devastating to her health. Sharon could have died during pregnancy.

The donor went on to the egg retrieval stage. Embryos were created with Sharon's partner's sperm. The embryos were then frozen and Sharon began her quest to look for a gestational carrier or surrogate mother to carry her baby because of her cardiac vulnerability.

Needless to say, if Sharon had completed her cardiac evaluation earlier in the process, it would have saved her a great deal of stress, and she could have had her baby sooner, as she had hoped.

Nurses and ancillary staff in infertility clinics have been known to cheer when their patients get positive pregnancy tests. They want to see positive outcomes and positive results for their patients. In fact, as mentioned earlier, many of the treatment team (nurses, sonographers, receptionists) are drawn to the infertility field because they've had personal experience with infertility and difficult pregnancies. It is important to remember even through stressful moments that your treatment team is on your side.

Infertility Treatment for the Mind and Spirit

Challenges and disappointments are inevitable during infertility treatment. Infertility threatens what you may have dreamed and envisioned for your future. Treatment centers all over the country have added counseling services because of the emotional stress experienced by infertility patients. We encourage you to take advantage of counseling offered by your clinic so that misdirected anger does not affect your treatment.

Stress can be a big factor in pregnancy. Dana and Jim had gone through three IVF cycles with another treatment center before coming to our clinic. During their initial consultation with us, this couple expressed fears but appeared to agree that they wanted to make another attempt to have a child through IVF. All went well with their workup and their stimulation cycle, but then Dana called one of our nurses with some sad news. She was on her eighth day of egg stimulation when Jim served her with divorce papers. Dana was devastated. "We were fighting about every day issues," she said. "We treated each other horribly, and the topic of infertility was not even what we seemed to be fighting about."

Stress over infertility concerns can affect every aspect of your life and your relationship. The wide range of emotions can overwhelm. We see patients experience hope and great excitement one moment, and then plunge into depression and grief the next. Patients have told us that they've burst into tears during business meetings because of pent-up emotions related to their infertility.

Grieving is often part of the process for patients dealing with infertility. It is normal to experience sadness and frustration. We encourage patients to prepare themselves for the emotional turbulence associated with infertility. Those emotions include shock, sadness, anger, obsessing over infertility, social withdrawal, depression, resentment, grief, and guilt. Understanding that these feelings are common will help you deal with them.

Suzanne came bursting into our clinic's lobby in a frenzy. "I'm late. I'm sorry. I just got my fifth speeding ticket in a month trying to get to my appointments on time."

Since she'd received five speeding tickets in just two months, Suzanne was ordered by the traffic court judge to attend traffic school. Even her traffic school instructor told her she needed to reduce the stress in her life. Suzanne was incredulous: "Do you really think so?"

The fact is that we have many infertility patients who need relief from the stress, whether they realize it or not. We created a mind-body program to help our patients, and many other clinics have instituted similar programs. The concern is that stress from infertility challenges can overwhelm you or harm your relationships at a time when you need to focus on your goal to start a family.

We encourage our patients to find an appropriate outlet to relieve frustrations and disappointments. Counseling can help reduce your stress, and so can exercise, yoga, and other activities that take your mind off infertility and get your cardiovascular system pumping. Take time to have fun with family and friends. Pursue activities or hobbies to give your mind a vacation from your fertility fight.

We have had patients who become so caught up in their infertility challenges that they become their own worst enemies. Monique, for example, was one of the most difficult patients we've had. She had apparently taken the "squeaky wheel" axiom way too seriously. But she didn't squeak. She screamed. She demanded. She harassed.

The primary nurse assigned to her case was no rookie, but she finally refused to work with Monique because of her rudeness and her self-centered demands. Our nurse manager stepped in. She explained to Monique that no one would work with her if she continued to scream at our staff.

Monique was contrite. "I don't mean to be like this, but this is all so stressful, and it is frustrating that no one calls me back."

"Would you call someone if you knew you were going to be screamed at?" the nurse manager asked.

Patients need to understand that your infertility treatment team members, like other human beings, want to be treated with respect. They also try to keep their own stress levels to a minimum. If you scream at them, they will schedule their conversations with you for the end of the day so that they can complete other tasks before being lambasted. It's no secret that nurses in hospitals and clinics everywhere learn to put the charts of difficult patients at the bottom of their to-do lists. They deal with them near day's end rather than ruin an entire shift.

Taking care of yourself is not always on the top of your daily to-do list because it is seen as a luxury or the easiest thing to let go of. Caring for yourself physically, mentally, emotionally, and spiritually is necessary for your well-being. Many patients turn to their faith to find comfort, and we encourage them to do that, too.

Effective Communication

Building an effective working relationship with your treatment team is essential; this can be achieved by understanding how the clinic works. Establishing ways to communicate will be essential to your success and will help you create a more positive experience. Talk with your nurse about the best way to communicate, whether by email or phone messaging, and the time of day that you can be available to discuss your treatment. Find out the clinics hours of operation, how to contact the staff, how phone messages are returned, how to contact the physician, how billing works, etc. Make certain you know the correct numbers to call. Plan for your daily phone call from the nurse, and have your questions ready. We find that those patients who write down their questions don't require multiple phone calls.

Being familiar with your clinic's operations and staff can save you—and the staff—a lot of grief. Steven came running into our clinic office at 5:30 one afternoon, visibly angry and upset. He and his wife, Sarah, had driven 60 miles during rush hour trying to get to us before closing. "We tried calling and the phones were off. We were out of medication. We thought you'd gone for the day!" he screamed. "Why didn't you answer the phone?"

The nurse responded that he had called after the phones were off, but if he'd listened to the answering message, he would have heard it provide an after-hours emergency number that he could have called to reach a nurse who would have helped him get the medication his wife needed—at a pharmacy near their home.

Steven was very upset because he feared the lack of medication would mess up his wife's entire IVF cycle. His angry outburst sent his wife running out of the clinic to her car in embarrassment. She feared the staff would tell them they were no longer allowed to be treated at the clinic.

Our staff gathered to console him as Steven broke down, telling them that this was the one part of the treatment where he could help his wife, and he feared he had failed. He was overwhelmed from the stress. Steven calmed down but he couldn't stop sobbing, as his anger turned to embarrassment at the scene he had caused.

The nurse finally held his hand and assured him that we had the medication for his wife and that she would be able to continue her IVF cycle. She then went to the parking lot and brought in Sarah and helped this anxious couple settle down and get what they needed.

If Sarah and Steven had read through the standard information packet that we provided them, they would have seen the number for the after-hours emergency line. They could have avoided a 60-mile drive and a very stressful situation for all of us. Infertility is stressful enough; planning ahead, making sure you have asked all of your questions, and making sure your needs are taken care of during the clinic's hours will help prevent unnecessary frustrations.

Getting Good Information

Patients often make the treatment process more complicated and intense because they've picked up bad information from someone they've met or a relative, or on the Internet. Unreliable information flows like a polluted river through the Internet and into the community of people seeking fertility treatments. We tell patients that it is important to read and to educate themselves, even though we try to provide all the information they need. At our clinic, we have notebooks with a vast amount of information for our patients and partners.

Infertility blogs on the Internet can be helpful, but some carry inaccurate and even potentially dangerous information. Reputable fertility clinics treat each patient as a unique case. There is no one treatment that suits all. So it is important to keep in mind that one blogger's solutions will not work for all patients. Advice meant to be helpful may not be accurate or up-to-date. Tests and treatments are designed for each patient's unique needs. You can't assume that a treatment touted by a blogger will work for you or your loved one. There are credible and helpful Web sites, including those for RESOLVE (www.resolve.org) and the American Society for Reproductive Medicine (www.asrm.org). These are good resources for patients to gain more reliable information. Those who serve on your treatment team are the best resources, so make an appointment if you have questions.

Flexibility and Fertility

We've given you a lot of guidance in this chapter and we hope it will be helpful. Stress management is very important as you undergo your treatments. Flexibility is also very important. That may not seem like a critical issue, but patients sometimes get locked into a very tight time frame for having a baby. Your treatment team may even buy into that goal and adopt it. But having a set date in your mind can be a setup for disappointment.

Remember that your treatment schedule is based on results of tests such as blood screening, ultrasounds, and urine samples, among others. Some tests are required to be completed on a specific day of your cycle, which may require you to complete that test next month. We often remind patients that although in vitro fertilization or artificial inseminations are treatments, they are also diagnostic, in that they give us our first look at things like your ovulation, the eggs' fertilization, and embryo quality. During your treatment, your team may discover issues or problems that create delays in the anticipated schedule or a change in the original plan. The disappointments of canceling a cycle and changing work, travel, and home schedules can feel enormous. That's why we encourage you to remain flexible and hopeful as your treatment team works for you and your dreams.

Chapter Nineteen

A Patient's Story

I've offered you patients' perspectives throughout this book, so here is one final story, that of Michelle and Thad Eldredge. Their opinions are their own. They had a long and arduous fight, and we hope you will benefit from their experience and insights.

Our Fertility Journey
Michelle Eldredge

So many things have shaped me as an individual, but nothing quite like my infertility journey. I grew up with a healthy work ethic. I was a good student, a gymnast for many years. I received an academic scholarship to college and went to graduate school. So, I thought if you work hard enough for what you want, it will come. My infertility story supports this notion that working hard will get you what you want, but I never knew work like this!

For some, the path to parenthood is a short story. Then, there is ours. My husband, Thad, and I tried to conceive naturally for about a year. I was 33 years old at the time and thought having a baby in the spring would be nice. Yeah, right!

After one year without getting pregnant, I met with my OB-GYN, and he carefully explained the sequence of events for conceiving a child. I like sequence and structure and control. So after we met and he gave me suggestions for some diagnostic fertility tests, I thought I'd become pregnant soon. *Not quite.*

I've formed many opinions about infertility treatment as the result of my experiences. These are a few of them, for what they are worth:

Opinion 1: Seek help and ask questions, especially as you approach your midthirties.

After my first visit with my OB-GYN, my first fertility diagnostic test was an HSG test. [HSG stands for *hysterosalpingogram*, an x-ray of the uterus and fallopian tubes.] This test came back normal (I would later learn this might not give you the best idea of the health of your uterus), but another test revealed that I was not ovulating, so I was prescribed Clomid. After my first unsuccessful month on Clomid, I had a gut feeling there was more going on than what Clomid could fix. I made a self-referral to a reproductive endocrinologist in Denver, Colorado. My only basis for choosing the doctor I did at the time was that they filed my health insurance (not a good reason). I was also becoming concerned that I was getting older, and I thought my fertility would be taking a nosedive at age 35.

Opinion 2: Not all reproductive endocrinologists are the same.

I had a one-hour meeting with my first reproductive endocrinologist (RE) by myself and heard a lot of the same information that my OB-GYN had explained to me, but he recommended a bit more testing. I had an ultrasound that revealed many small follicles. (That's good, but why so many and why so small? I would not find out about that until later.) They also found things that looked liked "holes" in my uterus.

The RE did not know what they were, but thought they might be fibroids, yet she said they were located in an area where a baby does not normally implant and told me not to worry about these "holes." (Again, red flag!)

My husband went in a week later for his sperm analysis. He was nervous but very willing to do what it took to help the process along. I then did three rounds of IUI (intrauterine insemination) with Clomid, increasing the dose of Clomid each month with no success. The only monitoring was an ultrasound checking to see if there was a "lead" follicle. I maybe, sort of, kind of, had a "lead" follicle each time. I was given the advice of waiting a couple of more days for this "lead" follicle to develop before the IUI was to happen.

My uterine lining was never checked, and there was never a repeat ultrasound to indeed check if the "lead" follicle was mature before each of my IUIs.

After my third failed IUI, the RE said I needed to go on Lupron to shrink my possible fibroid and then consider in vitro fertilization (IVF).

Opinion 3: Seek a second opinion.

I agreed to take the Lupron for one month, and before my second month of Lupron, I made my second self-referral—this time to Dr. Schoolcraft. My appointment with Dr. Schoolcraft was scheduled one day before my second Lupron shot was to happen.

Opinion 4: You get what you pay for.

While I was very fortunate to have infertility benefits through my employer, my new clinic did not accept my health insurance. However, I could file it on my own through my out-of-network benefit. By this point, I was willing to do anything and everything and spend the money it took to get pregnant. I was about to embark on countless hours of health insurance paperwork.

I had to be very organized about keeping receipts, filing my own medical insurance claim forms and keeping track of what, how much, and when I was getting reimbursed for the different doctor and diagnostic test visits. I still have my four accordion file folders full of just health insurance paperwork. At the end of my first visit with my new doctor, I paid for the doctor's fee, blood tests, and a $1,000 down payment to proceed with my first IVF cycle.

Here is what I found out upon my very first visit with my doctor:

○ I had 100 percent immunity to my husband's sperm.

○ I had fibroids.

○ I had adenomyosis, a painful condition in which tissue that normally lines the uterus also grows within the muscle walls of the uterus. My best chance of having a baby was IVF.

○ My fibroids would have to be removed.

○ My uterine blood flow number was elevated so I was referred for acupuncture.

Opinion 5: Go for acupuncture.

After my surgery to remove the fibroids, I met with a clinic nurse to learn how and when to give the shots for my IVF protocol. I was excited to get the process started. I was also reminded to visit an acupuncturist to help reduce my uterine blood flow, since that might hinder my chances of getting pregnant during an IVF cycle.

My acupuncturist and I became very close. She educated me on all things infertile and fertile and helped me maintain my sanity for the long journey ahead. I never felt more relaxed in my life than during those acupuncture treatments. It was truly the only time I could get my mind off of everything. Acupuncture also treated my elevated uterine blood flow to increase my chances of conceiving during our first IVF attempt.

Opinion 6: Great embryo quality does not mean you will become pregnant.

I was fortunate to respond very well to the stimulation medications and even "coasted" for a couple of days. (I was told not to take as much medication as my follicles were developing well, but they did not want them to develop too quickly.) I took my trigger shot and my doctor retrieved 25 eggs. By day 5, I had 10 embryos worthy of transfer. The two that were transferred even received the top grade possible. There was a brief conversation on transfer day about the option of only transferring one embryo, but we decided to transfer the top two embryos.

We waited about 10 days for our results. My hCG came back at a 1.5. [hCG stands for *human chorionic gonadotropin*. The level of this hormone present is an early indicator of pregnancy.] I was incredibly sad. I was sad for me, my husband, and the embryos that I'd hoped would be born 9 months later. I had not felt so sad since my father passed away, 5 years prior.

It was a beautiful fall day in the mountains of Colorado, and I remember thinking all of the awesome colors of the mountains became dull that day. They stayed dull for a long while. My husband was out of town and I lay in bed crying for the next 2 days.

Opinion 7: Be open to suggestions.

My husband and I scheduled a meeting to regroup with my doctor about 2 weeks after our failed first IVF attempt. I felt my life had already been consumed by infertility. I read every book, magazine, Web site, and blog imaginable on the subject. I gave up caffeine, chocolate, and alcohol, and I went to acupuncture twice a week. I felt infertility had put stress on my job, my friends, and my husband. It was hard to see the joy in anything.

I was consumed with trying to have a child. Why was this so hard? Why me? Why us? Why was this so time-consuming? Why was this so expensive—physically, emotionally, and financially?

I thought my doctor would just say it is a numbers game and we can try again with our 8 frozen embryos and have a good chance of getting a baby next time. I was wrong, very wrong. He said our IVF attempt failed for probably one of two reasons—an undiagnosed chromosomal problem, or my uterus.

My doctor suggested we start looking for a gestational carrier if we wanted to have our own biological children. He suggested first trying to find a family member or a friend before looking into an agency. My husband turned to me and said, "Kate."

My best friend from childhood is Kate, beautiful inside and out, healthy, outgoing, and incredibly loyal. My husband had digested what the doctor was saying much quicker than I had. *A gestational carrier?*

Our doctor explained the difference between a gestational carrier and a surrogate, something that would be very helpful to know later on in our infertility journey. But first, the doctor decided to once again have me try Lupron for 3 months to shrink the adenomyosis that was thought to be the probable cause of my failed IVF.

We could then proceed with one more attempt at a frozen cycle, and then think about going with a gestational carrier if this did not work, he said.

Still, I immediately called Kate to ask her to be our gestational carrier. I was in tears. She immediately said yes and we began talking for endless hours on the phone discussing what this all meant.

Opinion 8: Infertility treatment is a job.

Shortly after our first unsuccessful IVF attempt, I learned there was a good chance I would be laid off from my job and lose my health benefits along with the income I needed to help pay for upcoming treatments. I was stressed to my maximum, or so I thought. It did not help that the Lupron I was on caused me to forget words and to wake up many times during the night with hot flashes.

I was miserable. I did not like waiting to try to have another baby while the Lupron did its thing. I was not happy, and I know my husband was not too happy being around me. My world became very small. I could hardly stand to hear another woman talk about being pregnant. I could not go to a shopping mall because it seemed like every woman but me was pregnant.

I was fortunate to find another job. However, I also felt like infertility had become my job, and I did not like this job much.

Opinion 9: Find a support group.

I was fortunate that my clinic provided a support group for men and women going through infertility. I did not feel so alone in this process and came to realize instead of *Why me* I could say, *Well, why not me?* I learned some valuable information in these sessions and met some really great people. We all had our own journey and subsequently some very different infertility outcomes. Acupuncture also continued to help keep me somewhat sane.

Opinion 10: Continue to ask questions.

As I was waiting to go through our first frozen transfer, I had made an appointment to speak with a doctor at my clinic to follow up on a possible diagnosis of PCOS, or *polycystic ovary syndrome*. (Remember those many, albeit small, follicles I mentioned earlier?) PCOS patients produce a lot of small follicles but never ovulate and therefore have difficulty in conceiving a child. I learned the doctor specialized in the treatment of PCOS patients. It had been somewhat mentioned in the past that I might also have PCOS, but I had this insatiable urge to try to know everything possible before we tried again.

I was indeed diagnosed with PCOS, and we asked for chromosomal tests for my husband and me. (There is no connection between the two; I just wanted to have everything checked before we tried again.) I also asked for testing to see if I had a clotting problem that would prevent me from carrying a pregnancy. I wanted to know and do everything possible before the next try. As it turned out, I had PCOS but not a clotting problem. Our chromosomes were okay.

Opinion 11: Be patient, if and when you can.

After 3 months of Lupron, I was cleared to prepare for our first frozen embryo transfer. My first was cancelled because my uterine lining was not at least 8 millimeters in thickness. I was sad and mad and frustrated. I was in the throes of what I thought was hormone hell. I stopped my medications, got my period, and was told I could try again the next month with some more medication help to build up my lining.

The next month, I went back on estrogen patches and vaginal estrogen in combination with vaginal Viagra, and I continued acupuncture to build up my lining. It was not the most convenient protocol (I am not sure really any of them are), but it was working and my next frozen embryo attempt was scheduled. A couple of days before we were scheduled for a frozen embryo transfer, my grandmother passed away. We were able to delay our transfer for a few days as I traveled to say good-bye to my grandmother. I continued to think, how much more can I be tested?

Then, much to our surprise, our frozen transfer was a success, and I was pregnant—but only for about 10 weeks. I found out that I miscarried at my first OB appointment. This was my first visit with a new doctor on Dr. Schoolcraft's team, and I could tell she felt almost as bad as I did. I was in shock and numb. I called my husband to tell him the bad news and then went from the OB's office directly to the doctor's office. She reconfirmed by ultrasound that I had miscarried. This was a Friday. I was scheduled for a D&C the following Monday.

I called my best friend, Kate, on the way home from the doctor's office. She said the most amazing thing to me: "I have always been your backup." I cried almost the entire weekend. I started bleeding over the weekend and thought I might miscarry on my own, but was told to increase my previous dose of progesterone to try and stop that from happening. The hope of the D&C was to perform a chromosomal analysis on the embryo. I found out a couple of weeks later we were carrying a normal baby girl.

Opinion 12: Do not be too quick to judge others.

After my D&C, I needed to go in for a couple of blood tests to ensure that my hCG numbers were continuing to decline. Not fun. At one of these appointments, I saw a woman come into my doctor's office with a baby. I could not believe that someone could come into an infertility office with a baby! How dare she!

This woman would end up becoming a friend and playing an instrumental role in helping me navigate through the not-so-straight-forward gestational carrier process, as she had used a gestational carrier to have her son. She would give me the answer to one major hurdle: maternity insurance. Without health insurance coverage for a possible pregnancy, I did not think we could proceed using Kate as our carrier. Kate's health insurance policy specifically had an exclusionary clause about coverage for surrogacy pregnancies, which also meant no health insurance coverage for a gestational carrier pregnancy.

I could find no health insurance coverage in the state of North Dakota (where Kate lived) that would give Kate maternity coverage for a gestational carrier pregnancy. The woman I met in the doctor's office that day gave me my answer. There was an insurance company in California that specifically covered gestational carrier pregnancies. She gave me the information and we were on our way. I am forever grateful for our chance meeting.

Opinion 13: Give yourself a break.

I quit my new job of only 8 months after I miscarried. I needed to figure out all of the details of having a baby through a gestational carrier. I continued doing what I thought was my never-ending research and attended a couple of adoption meetings with my husband. I wanted to know there were alternatives and whether we would have a chance at being parents if this next huge step with Kate did not produce a child.

Kate is from Fargo, but she offered to come to Denver for her workup with our doctor. She arrived in Denver about 5 weeks after I miscarried. Before Kate could have her workup, the doctor wanted to see her medical history during her pregnancy with her daughter. Kate had her records sent and we embarked on the emotional, financial, and legal journey of what it meant to be a gestational carrier for both of our friends and family. I was so grateful to Kate for her commitment and support of our becoming parents.

Opinion 14: A gestational carrier is not a surrogate.

Using a gestational carrier is a unique experience, to say the least. It is an incredible gift, but it is expensive, and there are legal and emotional considerations to understand for all parties involved. Each state has its own legal opinions on surrogates and gestational carriers. A surrogate donates not only her body to carry a child but also her own egg. A gestational carrier donates her body to carry an embryo for the intended parents. It all came into clear focus as to why my doctor had made this important distinction to us months prior. All of this legal information made me a bit nervous, but we found an attorney (and a former gestational carrier) in North Dakota to help us through the process.

My husband, Kate, and I signed a very thorough legal agreement that would protect all of us through the process. If all went well, using a gestational carrier would probably cost us almost $100,000 between medical and insurance, costs, and compensation costs for our carrier. A week before I miscarried, we had sold our house. That would help us pay for all the expenses of using a gestational carrier.

Opinion 15: Keep trying.

We got the green light to proceed with the next round of IVF. Kate was cleared to be our carrier, we had the legal documents in place, we were granted a maternity health insurance policy for Kate, and we had the support of the very close and few people we told about what we were doing next on our quest to have a child.

Thad and I met with the genetic counselors to understand the PGD (*preimplantation genetic diagnosis*) process and how it might enhance our chances of having a healthy baby.

We choose to do fresh IVF cycle and decided to do PGD testing on the embryos from this cycle to increase our chances of transferring chromosomally normal embryos to Kate. My doctor had put me on metformin for the PCOS to enhance the quality of my follicles for this next IVF cycle. I continued acupuncture and prayed really hard. The doctor retrieved 29 eggs, performed the PGD testing on day 3, and Kate flew to Denver a couple of days after my retrieval to wait for the transfer.

Transfer day arrived, and I had come down with the flu the night before the transfer. I could hardly sit up from being sick the night before, and I was so nervous. We waited in the waiting room for Kate to have her pre-transfer acupuncture, and I came across an article in a magazine I was reading about being a "childless couple." I thought this was a sign and was pretty convinced we might all be wasting our time. I had become very cynical.

We went back for the transfer and found out that our previously frozen embryos and fresh embryos had all undergone the PGD testing. We learned that our frozen embryos were classified as "mosaics," and many of our fresh embryos had a variety of chromosomal abnormalities. We had five or six chromosomally normal embryos to work with; however, on day 5, the fresh embryos were supposed to have made it to the blastocyst stage, but the embryos that were candidates for transfer had only made it to the morula stage, which means they were acting more like day 4 embryos than day 5 embryos.

It seemed like this craziness would never end! We decided to transfer three embryos based on the genetic testing, the grading of the embryos, and recommendations from the doctor on how many to transfer. Kate was a trooper throughout this entire meeting. I remember looking at our embryos through the microscope and hardly being able to see them because I was crying. They looked like a bunch of grapes. We did the transfer and went back to a hotel in Denver for Kate to do her bed rest. I was still sick with the flu, and we both fell asleep for the night after an incredibly trying day.

Opinion 16: Letting go is good.

Kate is a high-energy person, so she was not enthused about the orders for bed rest. She did her best to remain still, and after 2 days, we left the hotel, went to lunch, and then to the airport to send her back to North Dakota. I was convinced that we once again had a failed attempt at having a child.

I again cried most of the way from the airport to our home in the mountains of Colorado for the dreaded wait until the pregnancy test. Kate told me the night before her pregnancy test that she was sure she was pregnant. I got off the phone with her and saw a story on the national news of a woman who had used a gestational carrier to get pregnant and found out 2 months later she was pregnant herself. Go figure. Must be nice.

Opinion 17: Take one day at a time.

Kate had her pregnancy test the first day of my new job. I was meeting with my new boss for the day, and as we were at lunch he was wondering why I would not eat anything. I had told him before I accepted the position of my unique situation and why I had to delay my start date, and so I think he understood the pressure I was undergoing that day. While we were at lunch, Kate called, but I had left my phone in our meeting room. My clinic had also called. My husband had also called. Kate had called my phone about nine times. I was shaking. I called Kate, and she said she was pregnant! I called and spoke with one of the clinic nurses, and she told me Kate had a very healthy hCG number and would need to take another test 2 days later to see whether her hCG number doubled. I called my husband—we were both excited but realistic about the days and hopefully the months ahead.

Kate went in for her second blood test on Christmas Eve 2006, and her number had almost tripled. What an amazing Christmas gift!

I was cautiously optimistic, but knew from previous experience that you need to take this process one day at a time. I was right. Kate started bleeding 3 days before her first ultrasound. I knew it; it was over. Another failure. I wanted to crawl out of my skin and be someone else. I could not take anymore disappointment. That day, my husband and I were moving my stuff into a new apartment I needed to have for my new job. It was a cold and dreary day. Kate was told to rest and see what the ultrasound showed the next week. The bleeding stopped after about a day. I was not relieved by this and was again convinced the pregnancy was over as soon as it started.

Opinion 18: Dreams do come true.

Kate went in for her first ultrasound at her OB's office in North Dakota and was told she was carrying a singleton pregnancy. It did provide some relief to know there was a heartbeat, but my cynical, self-preserving self was not convinced her pregnancy would continue.

Kate had been convinced all along she was carrying twins. She went in for her second ultrasound, at 8 weeks, which did reveal twins. She was right! Her 6-year-old daughter called me on the phone and said—which I will never forget—"My mommy is going to have two babies for you." I immediately asked her to put her mom on the phone. Yes, indeed, it was two, she said, and calmly said this explained why she was so tired and eating so much!

I called the company providing the maternity insurance for Kate and paid the premium for twins, which was about $5,000 more than for a singleton. I started to get excited.

From this point forward, Kate and I spoke almost every day to check in with one another. She had a great pregnancy. She ate healthfully, exercised, and took very good care of herself. I went to North Dakota to attend as many doctor appointments as I could. Kate found out we were having boy-girl twins at her 14-week appointment.

Kate owns her own personal training business and worked right up until the point she delivered the twins. She carried them to 38 weeks and delivered our son vaginally and our daughter by C-section after a long, at times very stressful, 13-hour labor. Kate returned to work after one week with strict orders to take it easy (difficult for her to do, but she did) and provided breast milk via daily frozen Fed-Ex shipments from North Dakota to Colorado for more than a month. The local paper in Fargo, North Dakota, published a story about our journey. My husband and I refused to let the story run in the paper until after the twins were born and we knew they and Kate had come through the birth process healthy.

Our son Samuel "Sam" James Eldredge was born at 8:52 p.m. on August 13, 2007. Our daughter Katherine "Kate" Elizabeth Eldredge was born at 9:02 p.m. on August 13, 2007.

Two awesome kids!

Michelle's Final Words of Advice

1. Trust your gut. If you are not pregnant after a year of trying, seek help. If you are over 35, seek help sooner. Do not wait.

2. Get a second opinion, or a third, if needed. Educate yourself on infertility.

3. Ask your doctor and others questions about fertility options.

4. Do not compare your infertility story to others. We each have our own stories and journeys.

5. Do not judge people's infertility decisions. You must do what is right for you and your family.

6. Be patient with yourself. Be angry, sad, resentful, thankful, and joyful when you need to be. You most likely will visit all of these emotions throughout the infertility process.

7. Do not always believe what you read or hear about infertility (except this book, of course!). Ask your doctor to provide you with the answers and guidance.

8. Find a support group or go to therapy. It is helpful to try and maintain a perspective on what you are going through. It will help you maintain that you are not losing your mind or control over your life.

9. Never say *never*. Move through the infertility process with an open mind. Expand your "personal bandwidth" for accepting recommendations from a trusted doctor.

10. Research what your health insurance will cover for infertility. It is an expensive process and you need to know what financial help is available. Ask you doctor if there are other payment options for treatment.

11. Remember that your spouse or significant other is going through infertility as well. Respect and listen to his or her feelings.

12. Seek to get the best treatment possible. Research the different infertility doctors. Understand their statistics.

13. If you have been given an infertility diagnosis, accept it and work around and with it as much as you can.

14. Let Western and Eastern medicine help you in getting pregnant.

15. Be open to the fact that it does take a village to raise a child, but it might also take a village to have a child.

16. Take one day at a time because that is all we have.

17. Thank the doctors, nurses, techs, and administrative staff for helping you on your journey. Ask them questions when you do not understand something, from billing to blood tests.

18. Respect your decision to have children or not to.

19. Do not feel the need to explain what you are going through if you do not feel like doing so.

20. If you are blessed to have children, appreciate and love them as much as possible.

Glossary

Ablation: Separation, detachment, removal or destruction of a part, especially by cutting.

Adenomyosis: A noncancerous invasion of endometrial tissue into the uterine muscle wall that can cause painful and heavy menstrual periods.

Adhesion: Scar tissue in the abdominal cavity, fallopian tubes, or inside the uterus that can interfere with egg transport and implantation of the embryo in the uterus.

Amenorrhea: The absence of menstruation.

Amniocentesis: A test in which amniotic fluid is aspirated to test the fetus for genetic abnormalities.

Androgens: Male androgens are produced by the testes and trigger body hair and other masculine characteristics, while female androgens are produced in both the adrenal glands and ovaries. In women, an excess of androgens might cause irregular periods, excessive body hair, obesity, and infertility.

Aneuploidy: An abnormal number of chromosomes.

Anovulation: The absence of ovulation.

Antibodies: Antibodies are usually chemicals made by the body's immune system to fight infections; however, sometimes the body gets tricked into making antibodies against itself. When they attack the sperm or a fetus, they can result in infertility.

Anticardiolipin antibodies (ACA): These may be associated with recurrent miscarriage, but not infertility.

Antigen: A substance that causes antibodies to form.

Antiphospholipid antibodies (APA): Doctors test for antiphospholipid antibodies to be sure that the immune system isn't targeting the embryo as a foreign body or invader, which would make conception difficult.

Antisperm antibodies (ASA): Both men and women can produce sperm antibodies that render sperm unable to fertilize an egg. Special tests are needed to detect this cause of infertility. Men who have had testicular infections, trauma, or surgeries such as vasectomies are particularly at risk for the presence of these antibodies.

Artificial insemination (AI): Also known as *intrauterine insemination* (IUI), this is a fertility-enhancing process in which sperm is washed and concentrated, then placed at the top of the uterus so that more sperm reaches the egg or eggs.

Asherman's Syndrome: The uterine walls adhere to each other, causing the risk for infertility and miscarriages, usually due to uterine inflammation.

Aspiration: A process for suctioning fluid, such as that inside a follicle, which is done to retrieve an egg.

Assisted hatching (AH, AZH): Thinning out the female egg's shell or *zona pellucida*, done before the transfer of an embryo into the uterus.

Assisted reproductive technology (ART): Umbrella name for procedures for causing conception when sexual intercourse is not working. These include intrauterine insemination, in vitro fertilization, gamete intrafallopian transfer, and zygote intrafallopian transfer.

Asthenozoospermia: Low sperm motility.

Asymptomatic: Lack of symptoms.

Autoimmune: An immune reaction against the body's own tissue.

Azoospermia: No sperm in the ejaculate.

Balanced translocation (BT): Occurs when genetic material (DNA) is exchanged between two different chromosomes. The parent still has the full complement of genetic material, so they are healthy. If just one abnormal chromosome is passed to the child, miscarriage may result. In rare cases, a child is born with this problem and faces significant medical issues.

Basal body temperature (BBT): The lowest point of a patient's body temperature, usually occurring early in the day. BBT is charted to predict ovulation, but fertility medications can throw off results.

Beta HCG test: Blood test to detect early pregnancies and to check embryonic development.

Bicornuate uterus: Congenital malformation of the uterus in which the upper portion, known as the "horn," is duplicated.

Blastocyst transfer: A process that allows embryos fertilized in vitro to reach the blastocyst stage before transferring them into the uterus.

Blastocyst: A 5-day-old embryo featuring two cell types and a central cavity.

Blastomere: A cell produced during cell division in the fertilized egg.

Blighted ovum: A fertilized egg attaches itself to the uterine wall but the embryo does not develop, causing a pregnancy to terminate very early.

Blood glucose (BG): Blood sugar.

Cervical mucus: The thick fluid in the cervix opening. Most of the time this "plug" keeps sperm and bacteria from entering the womb. At mid-menstrual cycle, the mucus thins out to allow sperm into the womb.

Cervix: The opening between the uterus and the vagina.

Chemical or biochemical pregnancy: A pregnancy confirmed by blood or urine tests but not visible on ultrasound because of a very early miscarriage. Also called preclinical pregnancy.

Chlamydia: A common, bacterial sexually transmitted disease that can result in pelvic inflammatory disease.

Chocolate cyst: A cyst in the ovary filled with old blood, also known as an endometrioma.

Chromosome analysis: See *Karyotyping*.

Chromosomes: The structures in the cell that carry genetic material such as genes or DNA. Most people have 46 chromosomes: 23 from the egg and 23 from the sperm.

Cilia: Tiny hairlike projections inside the fallopian tubes. These waving "hairs" effectively sweep the egg toward the uterus.

Cleavage: A series of cell divisions of the fertilized egg that form the blastomeres and transform a single-celled zygote into a multicellular embryo.

Clomid: Brand name for clomiphene citrate, a synthetic hormone that stimulates ovulation by tricking the body into releasing follicle-stimulating hormone (FSH), which aids conception.

Clomiphene citrate challenge test (CCCT, or Clomid challenge test): Entails taking 100 milligrams of clomiphene citrate on menstrual cycle days 5 to 9. Blood levels of FSH are measured on cycle day 3 and again on cycle day 10. Elevated blood levels of FSH on day 3 or day 10 are associated with low pregnancy.

Congenital adrenal hyperplasia: Enzymatic errors of metabolism in which there are deficient levels of enzymes involved in the synthesis of cortisol.

Conization: A procedure in which a cone-shaped section of the cervix is removed because of abnormal or precancerous cells.

Controlled ovarian hyperstimulation (COH or COS): The use of fertility medications to stimulate growth of multiple follicles for ovulation.

Corpus luteum: A gland that produces progesterone, which is responsible for preparing and supporting the uterine lining for implantation.

Cryopreservation: Fast freezing and storing process for sperm, embryos, and unfertilized eggs.

Cryopreserved: Freezing at a very low temperature to store embryos, eggs or sperm for future use.

Cryptorchidism: Undescended testicle(s).

Cumulus cells: Nutrient cells surrounding the egg.

Cumulus oophorus: Protective layer of cells surrounding the egg.

Cycle day: The first day of a woman's menstrual cycle, when full flow starts before midafternoon.

Cyst: A fluid-filled sac.

Cytomegalovirus (CMV): A group of viruses that cause cell enlargement in various organs. Infection in a fetus can cause jaundice, high-tone deafness, eye problems, malformation, or death.

Cytotoxin: An antibody or toxin that attacks the cells of particular organs.

D&C: See *Dilation and curettage.*

Danazol (Danocrine): A synthetic derivative of testosterone used to treat endometriosis. Side effects include oily skin, acne, weight gain, abnormal hair growth, deepening of the voice, and muscle cramps.

Day 1: The first day of a woman's cycle with menses in full flow (not just spotting). Flow should begin before midafternoon; otherwise the next day is considered Day 1.

Days post-ovulation (DPO): The number of days a woman is past ovulation. Counting begins the day after ovula-tion, so if ovulation is on Thursday, Sunday is considered 3 DPO.

Days post-transfer (DPT): The number of days a woman is past embryo transfer. Counting begins the day after transfer, so if is on Tuesday, Saturday would be 4 DPO.

DHEAS: See *Dihydroepiandrosterone sulfate.*

Diethylstilbestrol (DES): A synthetic estrogen compound administered in the late 1950s through 1970 to prevent preterm labor. It was found to cause abnormalities—classically a T-shaped uterus, which makes women susceptible to miscarriages. It was banned in 1971 by the US Food and Drug Administration.

Dihydroepiandrosterone sulfate (DHEAS): An androgen produced mostly by the adrenal gland.

Dilation and curettage (D&C): A procedure to diagnose and treat abnormal bleeding and to stop an unwanted pregnancy by dilating the cervical canal and scraping out the lining and contents of the uterus.

Donor egg: Egg from one woman "donated" to another facing infertility.

Donor insemination: Artificial insemination with donor sperm.

Dysmenorrhea: Painful periods.

Dyspareunia: Difficult or painful sex.

Ectopic pregnancy: A pregnancy that implants outside of the uterus, usually in the fallopian tube. If the tube ruptures or bleeds severely, this can be a serious medical problem.

EDC: Estimated date of confinement, or when the baby is due to be born.

Egg donation: The act of donating eggs to someone else for use in attempting pregnancy through in vitro fertilization.

Egg donor: A women who contracts to donate eggs to an infertile couple for in vitro fertilization.

Egg retrieval: Process for obtaining eggs from ovarian follicles with a special needle and ultrasound.

Egg: Also known as the *oocyte*, the female reproductive cell.

Ejaculate: Semen and sperm released at orgasm.

Elective abortion: The voluntary termination of a pregnancy for nonmedical reasons.

Embryo: Earliest stage of human development. Occurs after the sperm fertilizes the egg.

Embryo toxic factor (ETF): An immune response a woman may have against her own fetus that may result in the loss of the pregnancy. Treatment is high doses of progesterone until the 16th week of pregnancy.

Embryo transfer (ET): Placing an egg fertilized outside the womb into a woman's uterus or fallopian tube.

Endocrine gland: An organ that produces hormones.

Endocrine system: Glandular system including the hypothalamus, pituitary, thyroid, adrenals, and testicles or ovaries.

Endometrial biopsy (EB, Ebx, EMB): A test for *Luteal phase defect* or *Hyperplasia* during which the uterine lining is collected for analysis.

Endometrioma: A mass containing endometrial tissue and blood.

Endometriosis: Growth of endometrial tissue outside the uterus that may interfere with ovulation and with the implantation of the embryo.

Endometritis: An inflammation of the endometrium.

Endometrium: Inner lining of the uterus that grows and sheds in response to estrogen and progesterone stimulation. This bed of tissue nourishes an implanted embryo.

Endorphins: Natural narcotics in the brain that reduce sensitivity to pain and stress but may contribute to stress-related fertility problems.

Epididymis: A tubular organ on the testicle where sperm mature before leaving through the vas deferens.

Epididymitis: An inflammation of the epididymis.

Estimated due date (EDD): The approximate date set for birth.

Estradiol: Primary estrogen produced by the ovary that aids formation of the female secondary sex characteristics and supports the growth of the follicle and the development of the uterine lining.

Estrogen: Female sex hormone produced by the ovaries and responsible for stimulating the uterine lining to thicken during the first half of the menstrual cycle, in preparation for ovulation and possible pregnancy. A small amount of estrogen is also produced in the male when testosterone is converted to estrogen.

Fallopian tubes: Ducts in which eggs travel to the uterus upon release from the follicle. Sperm normally meet the egg in the fallopian tube, where fertilization usually occurs.

Fasting blood glucose (FBG): Blood glucose levels measured after not eating or drinking anything other than water overnight. Normally, the level is under 110. A reading over that level indicates impaired glucose tolerance or insulin resistance.

Fasting blood insulin: Insulin levels taken after not eating or drinking anything other than water overnight. Insulin is a hormone that breaks down sugar.

Fertility microscope: A small microscope to view saliva or cervical mucus.

Fetus: A baby between 8 weeks and term.

Fibroid: A benign tumor of the uterine muscle and connective tissue.

Fimbria: Fingerlike projections at the end of the fallopian tube nearest the ovary. During ovulation, these push the egg into the tube.

Fimbrioplasty: Surgery to repair damaged fimbria that may block the fallopian tubes.

Follicle-stimulating hormone (FSH): Pituitary hormone that stimulates sperm and follicle development. In the man, FSH stimulates cells in the testicles and supports sperm production. In the woman, FSH stimulates ovarian follicle growth. Elevated FSH levels indicate gonadal failure in both men and woman.

Follicle: Fluid-filled sac in the ovary that contains an egg released at ovulation.

Follicular phase: The pre-ovulatory phase of a woman's cycle.

Frozen embryo transfer (FET): A procedure where frozen embryos are thawed and placed into the uterus.

FSH: See Follicle-stimulating hormone.

Gamete intrafallopian transfer (GIFT): An alternative to in vitro fertilization for women with healthy tubes. After egg retrieval, the eggs are mixed with sperm and injected into the fallopian tubes. The procedure is done through laparoscopy.

Gamete: A reproductive cell; sperm in men and the egg in women.

Gestation sac: The fluid-filled sac where the fetus grows and develops.

Gestation: Period of fetal development in the uterus from implantation to birth.

Gestational carrier: A woman who carries a pregnancy for the genetic parents.

Gestational diabetes: A temporary inability to process sugar during pregnancy.

Gestational surrogate: A woman who agrees to be implanted with the egg of another woman to conceive using the intended father's sperm and assisted reproductive techniques. Unlike tradi-

tional surrogate mothers, the gestational surrogate is not the biological mother.

Glucola: A sugary drink used in glucose tolerance tests.

Glucose tolerance test (GTT): Screening test for insulin resistance, diabetes, and gestational diabetes.

GnRH: See *Gonadotropin releasing hormone.*

Gonadotropin releasing hormone (GnRH): Hormone that controls production and release of gonadotropins.

Gonadotropins: Hormones that control reproductive function.

Gonads: Glands that make reproductive cells and "sex" hormones. The male testicles make sperm and testosterone, and the female ovaries make eggs and estrogen.

Gonal-F: A genetically engineered, highly pure form of human follicle stiumlating hormone (FSH), which is responsible for stimulating the production of egg-containing follicles in women and sperm in men.

Gonorrhea: Sexually transmitted bacterial disease that may cause infertility

hCG/HCG: See *Human chorionic gonadotropin.*

Heparin: Blood thinner that prevents blood clots from forming.

Hirsutism: Overabundance of body hair in women with excess androgens.

hMG, HMG: See *Human menopausal gonadotropin.*

Hormone replacement therapy (HRT): Procedure to replace estrogen and progesterone in menopausal women.

Hormone: Substance produced by an endocrine gland.

HRT: See *Hormone replacement therapy.*

HSG: See *Hysterosalpingogram.*

Human chorionic gonadotropin (hCG): Hormone produced in early pregnancy that regulates the corpus luteum producing progesterone. This is injected to trigger ovulation in some fertility treatments. Also used in men to increase testosterone production.

Human menopausal gonadotropins: Combination of the hormones FSH and LH extracted from the urine of postmenopausal women and used to induce ovulation in fertility treatment.

Hydrosalpinx: Blocked, dilated, fluid-filled fallopian tube.

Hyperglycemia: High blood sugar.

Hyperinsulinemia: Overproduction of insulin.

Hyperplasia: Thickening of the endometrium that can lead to abnormal, precancerous cells.

Hyperprolactinemia: Condition in which the pituitary gland secretes too much prolactin that might suppress LH and FSH production, reduce male sex drive, and hamper ovarian function.

Hyperstimulation (Ovarian hyperstimulation syndrome, OHSS): Potentially life-threatening side effect of ovulation induction with injectable fertility medications such as hMG.

Hyperthyroidism: Overproduction of thyroid hormone that increases metabolism and "burns up" estrogen so rapidly that it interferes with ovulation.

Hypoestrogenic: Lower than normal levels of estrogen.

Hypoglycemia: Low blood sugar.

Hypoplastic uterus: An underdeveloped uterus.

Hypospermatogenesis: Low sperm production.

Hypothalamus: The brain's hormonal regulation center that secretes GnRH every 90 minutes or so, enabling the pituitary gland to secrete LH and FSH, which stimulate the gonads.

Hypothyroidism: Thyroid gland produces too little thyroid hormone, negatively affecting fertility by causing a lower sex drive and high prolactin in men and elevated prolactin and estrogen in women.

Hysterectomy: Surgery to remove the uterus and sometimes the cervix.

Hysterosalpingogram (HSG): X-ray of the pelvic organs in which a dye is injected through the cervix into the uterus and fallopian tubes to check for malformations of the uterus and blockage of the fallopian tubes.

Hysteroscopic myomectomy: A procedure in which the doctor removes a uterine fibroid while using a hysteroscope.

Hysteroscopy (HSC): Test for uterine abnormalities using a fiber-optic device. Minor surgical repairs can be done during the procedure.

ICI: See *Intracervical insemination.*

ICSI: See *Intracytoplasmic sperm injection.*

Immunosupressive drug: Medication that interferes with the normal immune response.

Immunotherapy: Treatment for an immune system disorder in which donor white blood cells are transfused into a patient who has recurrent miscarriages.

Implantation: Embedding of the embryo into tissue to access the mother's blood supply for nourishment, usually 5 to 10 days after ovulation.

In vitro fertilization (IVF): A fertility enhancing technique in which fertilization takes place outside the body, in a small glass dish.

Inhibin-B: A hormone that interferes with activity of the follicle-stimulating hormone.

Insulin: Hormone that controls blood sugar (glucose). Overproduction of insulin in relation to glucose can lead to weight gain and ovulation difficulties.

Intracervical insemination (ICI): Artificial insemination that deposits sperm into the cervical canal.

Intracytoplasmic sperm injection (ICSI): Procedure to inject a single sperm into the egg to fertilize, despite low sperm counts or nonmotile sperm.

Intrauterine growth retardation (IUGR): Reduced fetal growth caused by infection, inadequate placenta, or exposure to environmental or chemical toxins.

Intrauterine insemination (IUI): Artificial reproductive procedure that deposits washed sperm directly into the uterus, bypassing cervical mucus and putting it close to the fallopian tubes.

Intravaginal culture (IVC): Eggs and sperm are combined in a capsule and inserted into a woman's vagina to incubate for 48 hours so that fertilization can happen within the woman's body. After 24 hours, resulting embryos are transferred into the uterus.

Intravenous immunoglobulin (IVIg): Intravenous transfer of antibodies used for some immune problems.

IUI: See *Intrauterine insemination.*

IVC: See *Intravaginal culture.*

IVF: See *In vitro fertilization.*

Karyotyping: Chromosome analysis of cells for abnormalities.

Klinefelter's Syndrome: Genetic abnormality characterized by having one Y (male) and two X (female) chromosomes or a combination of 46XY and 47XX. Klinefelter's often causes a fertility problem, though some men will produce sperm.

Laparoscopic myomectomy: Removal of uterine fibroid using a long, narrow fiber-optic instrument called a laparoscope, which is inserted into a hole in the abdominal wall. A laparoscope can be used to diagnose and treat fertility prob-

lems including endometriosis, abdominal adhesions, and polycystic ovaries.

Laparoscopy: Surgery that allows viewing of the internal pelvic organs using a long, narrow fiber-optic instrument, called a laparoscope, which is inserted through an incision in or below the woman's navel. Other incisions may be made for inserting additional instruments.

Laparotomy: Major surgery to restore fertility, such as tubal repairs and the removal of adhesions or fibroids.

Leukocyte antibody detection assay (LAD): Test of a woman's physical response to pregnancy. Women with high levels of leukocyte antibodies may carry pregnancies longer than those with low levels. Women with low levels of leukocyte antibodies may have pregnancies that end by week 12, or their immune systems may not respond to the stimulus of pregnancy by creating blocking antibodies. Women with low levels of LAD are candidates for immunization with their husbands' white blood cells.

Leukocyte immunization therapy (LIT): Injecting a woman with her husband's or a donor's white blood cells to increase fetal blocking antibodies and lower her natural killer cells that keep the immune system in balance.

Leukocytosis: Increase in the number of leukocytes (white blood cells) generally caused by infection.

Leydig cell: Testicular cell that produces testosterone.

LH: See *Luteinizing hormone.*

Lupron: Injectable medication to regulate the pituitary gland and prevent release of substances such as LH and FSH. Without LH or FSH, the ovary will not produce follicles that will in turn decrease the production of estrogen and progesterone.

Luteal phase defect (or Luteal phase deficiency) (LPD): Occurs when the uterine lining does not develop because of inadequate progesterone stimulation, or because of the inability of the uterine lining to respond to progesterone stimulation. LPD may prevent embryonic implantation or cause an early miscarriage.

Luteal phase: Post-ovulatory phase of a woman's cycle. The corpus luteum produces progesterone that causes the uterine lining to thicken and support the implantation and growth of the embryo.

Luteinized unruptured follicle syndrome (LUFS): A condition in which the follicle develops and changes into the corpus luteum without releasing the egg. Use of anti-inflammatory drugs such as Advil, Motrin, and Aleve near ovulation may contribute to LUFS.

Luteinizing hormone (LH): Pituitary hormone that stimulates the gonads. In the man, LH is necessary for sperm development and for production of testosterone. In women, LH is necessary for production of estrogen. When estrogen reaches a critical peak, the pituitary releases a surge of LH, which releases the egg from the follicle.

Luteinizing hormone surge (LH Surge): Spike in the release of LH that causes release of a mature egg from the follicle. Ovulation test kits detect the sudden increase of LH, signaling that ovulation is about to occur (usually within 24 to 36 hours).

Lymphocytes: Cells present in the blood and lymphatic tissue that travel from the blood and lymph nodes and back into circulation. Lymphocytes are derived from the stem cells, from which all blood cells arise.

Menarche: A woman's first menstruation.

Menopause: End of menstruation in the female life cycle.

Menorrhagia: Heavy or prolonged menstrual flow.

Metrodin: An injectable follicle-stimulating hormone used to stimulate ovulation.

Micromanipulation: IVF lab process that holds eggs or embryos with special instruments to do procedures such as ICSI, assisted hatching, or embryo biopsy.

Microsurgical epididymal sperm aspiration (MESA): Microsurgery to remove sperm from the epididymis for in vitro fertilization.

Molar Pregnancy: Fertilization of an egg without a nucleus.

Morphology: Shape of sperm studied in a semen analysis.

Motility: Measure of motion and progression of sperm in a semen analysis.

Mutagen: Substance that alters the sperm or egg's genetic structure before conception.

Mycoplasma: Small bacteria-like organisms suspected of causing several urologic, obstetric, and gynecologic disorders, including pelvic inflammatory disease, urethritis, and pregnancy loss. Women whose reproductive tracts are colonized with Mycoplasma can have higher rates of miscarriage. The organism lives in the male prostate gland and is transmitted during intercourse.

Myomectomy: Surgical removal of uterine fibroids.

Natural killer cells: Cells that fight, kill and destroy their targets. Excessive numbers may result in pregnancy loss and reduced success in IVF cycle outcome.

Necrospermia: Sperm are produced but die in the semen.

Non-obstructive azoospermia: Impaired or nonexistent sperm production.

Nonsurgical sperm aspiration (NSA): A small needle is used to extract sperm directly from the testis in those who have blocked ducts or cannot ejaculate.

Obstructive azoospermia: Blockage in the male reproductive tract. Sperm production may be normal but the sperm are trapped inside the epididymis.

Oligomenorrhea: Infrequent menstrual periods.

Oligo-ovulation: Infrequent ovulation, usually less than six ovulations per year.

Oligospermia: Few sperm.

Oocyte: The female reproductive cell or egg.

Oophorectomy: Surgical removal of the ovaries.

Ovarian cyst: Fluid-filled sac inside the ovary that may be related to ovulation disorders, tumors of the ovary, and endometriosis.

Ovarian drilling: A procedure in which an electrosurgery needle is used to burn small holes into each ovary to reduce androgen levels and restore cycles in women with polycystic ovaries.

Ovarian failure: Failure of the ovary to respond to FSH stimulation from the pituitary because of damage or malformation of the ovary.

Ovarian hyperstimulation syndrome (OHSS): See Hyperstimulation.

Ovarian wedge resection: Surgical removal of a wedge of a polycystic ovary to aid ovulation.

Ovary: Female gonad that produces eggs and female hormones.

Ovulation induction: Performed to start ovulation.

Ovulation: Release of the egg from the ovarian follicle.

Ovum: The egg or reproductive cell from the ovary that contains the woman's genetic information.

Pap smear: Removal of cells from the cervix surface for study.

Partial zona dissection (PZD): A predecessor to ICSI in which the *zona pellucida*, or shell of an egg, is opened with either chemicals or a sharp instrument to allow easier access for sperm.

Paternal leukocyte immunization (PLI): Injecting a woman with the male partner's white blood cells to increase fetal blocking antibodies and lower natural killer cells.

PCO, PCOD, PCOS: See *Polycystic ovary syndrome.*

Pelvic inflammatory disease (PID): Infection of the pelvic organs that causes severe illness, high fever, and extreme pain. PID may lead to tubal blockage and pelvic adhesions.

Percutaneous epididymal sperm aspiration (PESA): A small needle is passed directly into the head of the epididymis and fluid is aspirated. Any sperm found are used with in vitro fertilization with ICSI.

Pergonal (hMG): Medication used to replace the pituitary hormones LH and FSH to induce ovulation in women who do not respond to clomiphene citrate. Often used for women who do not produce estrogen because of a pituitary gland or hypothalamic malfunctions. May also be given to men to stimulate sperm production.

Perinatologist: A doctor specializing in treating the fetus/baby and mother during pregnancy, labor, and delivery.

Placenta: Embryonic tissue that implants in the uterine wall and allows exchange of the baby's carbon dioxide and waste products for the mother's nutrients and oxygen via the umbilical cord.

Polycystic ovary syndrome (PCO, PCOD, or PCOS): Excessive production of androgens (male sex hormones) and the presence of cysts in the ovaries. Symptoms may or may not include excessive weight gain, acne and excessive hair growth, lack of ovulation, and irregular menses.

Polyp: Growth or tumor, usually benign, on an internal surface such as the uterine wall.

Polyspermy: More than one sperm enters and fertilizes an egg.

Post-coital test (PCT): Examination of the cervical mucus performed after intercourse to measure compatibility between the woman's mucus and the man's semen.

Post-testicular system: Ducts that store and deliver the sperm to the opening of the penis, including the glands that produce seminal fluids.

Preclinical pregnancy: Early pregnancy loss before the next period is due. Also called *chemical pregnancy.*

Pre-embryo: The fertilized egg before cell division.

Premature ovarian failure (POF): Halting of menses associated with high levels of gonadotropins and low levels of estrogen before age 40.

Premature rupture of membranes (PROM): Spontaneous rupture of fetal membranes at least 1 hour before the onset of labor, marked by fluid from the vagina.

Premenstrual syndrome (PMS): Emotional and physical disturbances after ovulation and prior to menstruation.

Pretesticular system: Male hormonal system responsible for stimulating sperm production and development of male secondary sex characteristics.

Progesterone: Hormone produced by the corpus luteum during second half of a woman's cycle. It thickens the lining of the uterus to prepare it to accept implantation of a fertilized egg.

Prolactin: Hormone that stimulates production of milk in breastfeeding women. High prolactin levels when not breastfeeding may result in infertility.

Prostaglandins: Hormone-like substances found in men and women.

Prostate gland: Gland encircling the male urethra that produces one-third of the fluid in semen.

Pyospermia: White cells in the semen that may indicate infection and/or inflammation.

Qualitative hCG test: A pregnancy test, such as a home pregnancy test, that gives a yes or no answer.

Quantitative hCG test: A pregnancy test in which the units of hCG are measured.

Recombinant follicle-stimulating hormone (R-FSH, R-hFSH): Genetically engineered follicle-stimulating hormone, unlike FSH extracted from the urine of postmenopausal women. Brand names are Gonal-F and Follistim.

Recurrent pregnancy loss (RPL): Repeated miscarriages.

Reproductive endocrinology: Medical specialty combining obstetrics and gynecology with endocrinology to treat reproductive disorders.

Reproductive immunology: Medical specialty combining obstetrics and gynecology with immunology to treat reproductive disorders related to immune problems.

Repronex (hMG): Medication to replace the pituitary hormones LH and FSH, to induce ovulation in women who do not respond to clomiphene citrate. Often given to women who do not produce estrogen because of a pituitary gland or hypothalamic malfunction. May be used to stimulate male sperm production.

Resistant ovary: An ovary that cannot respond to the follicle-stimulating message sent by FSH.

Retrograde ejaculation: Male fertility problem in which sperm travels into the bladder instead of out of the penis, due to a failure in the sphincter muscle at the base of the bladder.

Retroperitoneal: Refers to the area outside or behind the tissue that lines the abdominal wall.

Retroverted uterus: A condition in which the uterus is tilted back toward the rectum.

Rh factor: Genetically determined antigens in the red blood cells that can induce immunologic reactions. Some women develop a sensitization to Rh during pregnancy. If a woman is Rh negative and the male is Rh positive, she is a candidate for Rh incompatibility problems.

Rhogam (Anti-D): Immunization for Rh-negative women after a miscarriage, stillbirth, or live birth to prevent production of antibodies in any Rh-positive babies they may have in future pregnancies.

Salpingectomy: Surgical removal of the fallopian tubes.

Salpingitis isthmica nodosa: Fallopian tube abnormality in which the tube attaches to the uterus; characterized by nodules.

Salpingitis: Inflammation of fallopian tubes.

Salpingolysis: Surgery to remove adhesions restricting movement and function of reproductive organs.

Salpingo-oophorectomy: Surgery to remove fallopian tubes and ovaries.

Salpingostomy: Incision made in a fallopian tube to repair a tube or to remove an ectopic pregnancy.

Scrotum: Bag of skin and thin muscle surrounding the man's testicles, epididymis, and vas deferens.

Secondary infertility (SI): Inability of a couple to achieve a second pregnancy.

Secondary sex characteristics: Physical qualities that distinguish man and woman, such as beard, large breasts, and deep voice, as a result of sexual maturity.

Semen: Ejaculate fluid containing sperm and secretions from the testicles, prostate, and seminal vesicles.

Seminal vesicles: Pouchlike glands at the base of the bladder that produce much of the semen volume, including fructose for nourishing the sperm and a chemical that causes the semen to coagulate on entering the vagina.

Seminiferous tubules: Network of tubes in the testicles in which the sperm are formed, mature, and move toward the epididymis.

Septate uterus: Uterus divided into right and left halves by a wall of tissue that can cause an increased chance of early pregnancy loss.

Septum: A dividing wall within a body cavity, such as the wall dividing the uterus in half.

Serophene: Brand name for clomiphene citrate.

Sertoli (nurse) cells: Testicular cells that provide nourishment to immature sperm.

Sheehan's syndrome: Caused by profuse hemorrhage at the time of delivery. Severe blood loss shocks the pituitary gland, which dies and becomes nonfunctional.

SHG: See *Sonohysterogram*.

Short luteal phase: See *Luteal phase defect*.

Slow responder: A patient who takes longer than average (10 days) to produce mature follicles on injectable fertility medications.

Sonohystogram: Ultrasound or sonogram in which saline is injected into the uterus to check for abnormalities but does not require iodine dye injection or radiation.

Sperm agglutination: Sperm clumping caused by antibody reactions or infection.

Sperm bank: Storage for frozen sperm used in artificial insemination.

Sperm count: The number of sperm in ejaculate. Also called sperm concentration or sperm density; the number of sperm per milliliter.

Sperm maturation: Process during which sperm grow and gain their ability to swim; usually about 90 days.

Sperm morphology: Semen analysis that indicates the number or percentage of normal sperm in the sample. The higher the percentage of misshapen sperm, the less likely fertilization can take place.

Sperm motility: Ability of sperm to swim. Poor motility means sperm have difficulty reaching the egg.

Sperm penetration assay (SPA): Test of sperm's ability to penetrate a hamster egg stripped of the outer membrane; also called a "hamster test."

Sperm penetration: Ability of the sperm to penetrate the egg during fertilization.

Sperm washing: Laboratory process for separating sperm from semen, and separating motile sperm from nonmotile sperm. Used in assisted reproduction.

Spermatic cord: Cord that suspends the testes within the scrotum.

Spermatogenesis: Sperm production in the seminiferous tubules.

Stein-Leventhal disease: Another name for polycystic ovary syndrome.

Stem cells: Cells from which other types of cells can develop.

Stimulated cycle oocyte retrieval: A procedure in which the ovaries are stimu-

lated with medications such as hMG or pure FSH in the doctor's office. The eggs are removed by ultrasound aspiration from the ovaries. The eggs are mixed with sperm, placed in a small plastic dish, and left in the incubator for 2 days. The fertilized eggs are then transferred to the uterus through a small plastic catheter.

Superovulation: Use of fertility medications to stimulate growth of multiple follicles for ovulation. Also known as *controlled ovarian hyperstimulation* (COH).

Surrogate mother: A traditional surrogate mother agrees to use her eggs and the intended father's sperm to conceive via artificial insemination. In the traditional surrogacy, she is the biological mother but agrees to give up her rights to the child.

Synarel: Synthetic hormone to treat endometriosis or for regulation before or during a controlled ovarian hyperstimulation cycle.

Teratogen: Any substance capable of causing malformations in a developing embryo.

Testes: Two male sexual glands contained in the scrotum. They produce the male hormone testosterone and the sperm.

Testicle: Male gonad that produces sperm and male sex hormones.

Testicular biopsy: Minor surgical procedure to take a sample of testicular tissue for examination to diagnose male fertility problems.

Testicular enzyme defect: Congenital enzyme defect that prevents the testes from responding to hormonal stimulation and results in oligospermia or azoospermia.

Testicular failure: The primary form of this condition is a congenital, developmental, or genetic error resulting in a testicular malformation that prevents sperm production. The secondary form is testicular damage from drugs, prolonged exposure to toxic substances, or a varicocele.

Testicular stress pattern: Semen analysis result showing depressed sperm production, poor sperm motility, and poor sperm morphology.

Testicular torsion: A testicle twists on itself, cutting off its own blood supply and causing extreme pain.

Testosterone: Male hormone responsible for the formation of secondary sex characteristics and for supporting the sex drive; also necessary for sperm development.

Therapeutic abortion: Termination of a pregnancy due to severe abnormalities in the fetus or if the mother's health is at risk.

Thyroid gland: Endocrine gland in the front of the neck that produces thyroid hormones to regulate the body's metabolism.

Thyroid releasing hormone (TRH): Peptide hormone synthesized in the hypothalamus and passed through the hypophyseal portal venous system. In the anterior pituitary, TRH stimulates synthesis and release of thyroid stimulating hormone, or TSH.

Thyroid stimulating hormone (TSH): Also called thyrotropin, this hormone produced by the pituitary gland promotes growth of the thyroid gland and stimulates it.

Thyroxine: Chemical substance made by the thyroid gland, which uses iodine to make thyroid hormones. Thyroid hormones regulate growth and the rate of chemical reactions in the body.

Tipped uterus: A uterus tipped toward a woman's back instead of tilting forward.

Total effective sperm count: Estimate of the number of sperm in an ejaculate sample capable of fertilizing an egg.

Transvaginal ultrasound: Examination performed by inserting a probe into the vagina. This type of ultrasound is common for viewing follicle growth and can produce better images in early pregnancy than might be obtained with conventional sonograms.

Transvaginal: Through the vagina or across its wall.

Tubal embryo transfer (TET): Placement of an embryo inside the fallopian tube after in vitro fertilization.

Tubal ligation: Surgical sterilization by obstructing or tying the fallopian tubes.

Tubal patency: Open and unobstructed fallopian tubes.

Tubocornual anastomosis: Surgery to remove a blocked portion of the fallopian tube and to reconnect the tube to the uterus.

Tuboplasty: Plastic or reconstructive surgery on the fallopian tubes to correct abnormalities causing infertility.

Tubotubal anastomosis: Surgery to remove a diseased or damaged portion of the fallopian tube and reconnect the two ends; a sterilization reversal.

Turner's syndrome: The most common genetic defect contributing to female fertility problems, in which the ovaries fail to form.

Umbilical cord: Two arteries and a vein wrapped in a gelatinous tube leading from the baby to the placenta, which exchanges nutrients and oxygen from the mother for waste products from the baby.

Undescended testicles: Failure of the testicles to descend from the abdominal cavity into the scrotum by 1 year of age. If not repaired by age 6, this may result in permanent fertility loss.

Unexplained infertility: When the cause for infertility has not been determined.

Unicornate uterus: Abnormality in which the uterus is "one sided" and smaller than usual.

Ureaplasma: Infection that may cause formation of sperm antibodies and an inflammation of the uterine lining, both may interfere with implantation of the embryo.

Urethra: Tube that allows urine to pass between the bladder and the outside of the body. In males, this tube carries semen from the area of the prostate to the outside.

Urologist: A physician/surgeon specializing in the urinary tract and male reproductive tract.

Uterus: Hollow, muscular female reproductive organ that houses and nourishes the fetus during pregnancy; the womb.

Vagina: The female organ of sexual intercourse; the birth canal.

Vaginal ultrasound: Ultrasound imaging of the female reproductive system through an ultrasound device inserted into the vagina.

Vaginismus: Spasm of muscles around the opening of the vagina, making penetration during sexual intercourse impossible or painful.

Vaginitis: Inflammation of the vagina that may indicate presence of pelvic adhesions and tubal blockage from other infections, such as Chlamydia. Vaginitis can interfere with sperm penetration of the cervical mucus. The symptoms may even interfere with the ability and desire to have intercourse.

Varicocele: Varicose veins in the scrotum create a pool of stagnant blood, which elevates the scrotal temperature and causes male infertility.

Vas deferens: Pair of thick-walled tubes through which the sperm move from the epididymis to the ejaculatory duct in the prostate. These tubes are severed during a vasectomy.

Vasectomy reversal: Surgical repair of vasectomy to restore fertility.

Vasectomy: Surgical separation of both vas deferens for birth control and sterilization.

Vasogram: An X-ray of the vas deferens.

Venereal disease: Sexually transmitted infection, such as Chlamydia, gonorrhea, and syphilis. Many of these diseases will interfere with fertility, and some cause severe illness.

Viscosity: The thickness of semen.

Vulva: Woman's external genitalia.

X chromosome: Congenital, developmental, or genetic information in the cell that transmits the information necessary to make a female. All eggs contain one X chromosome, and half of all sperm carry an X chromosome. When two X chromosomes combine, the baby will be a girl.

Y chromosome: Genetic material that transmits the information necessary to make a male. Y chromosomes can be found in one-half of the man's sperm cells. When an X and a Y chromosome combine, the baby will be a boy.

Zona pellucida: Protective outer membrane surrounding the egg.

Zygote intrafallopian transfer (ZIFT): A procedure in which eggs are removed from a woman's ovaries and fertilized with the man's sperm in a lab dish, and the resulting fertilized eggs are transferred into the woman's fallopian tubes during a minor surgical procedure.

Zygote: Fertilized egg which has not yet divided.

ACKNOWLEDGMENTS

IT TAKES AN entire clinic of medical professionals to write a book of this scope. I would not have been able to complete this book without the collective efforts of many contributors. First, I would like to thank my fellow physicians, medical scientists, psychologists, therapists, counselors, and health care professionals who contributed their expertise to this comprehensive work.

The following CCRM team members each contributed substantially to the book, and I am grateful for all of the time, effort, and knowledge they put into this project.

Dr. Laurie J. McKenzie (basics of fertility treatment, miscarriages).

Dr. Debra Minjarez (polycystic ovarian syndrome, gestational carrier)

Dr. Eric Surrey (endometriosis, tubal and uterine challenges)

Dr. Timothy Hickman (in vitro fertilization, unexplained infertility)

Dr. Barrett Cowan (male infertility)

Dr. Robert L. Gustofson (donor sperm, egg donation and preservation, fertility protection)

Mandy Katz-Jaffe, PhD (genetic testing)

Kelly Lehl, RN, Debbie Levy, MA, LPC, and Alison J. Wilson, PhD (working with your fertility team, the emotional challenges of infertility)

Randine Lewis, PhD (alternative medicine)

I would like to give special thanks to all of our patients who shared their stories, especially Michelle Eldredge and her husband, Thad, and also to Debra Roth, the assistant practice administrator at CCRM, who coordinated the flow of information and materials and skillfully handled the many complex details that went into producing this book.

All of the contributions from our team were melded together and polished courtesy of the brilliant writing skills of my collaborator, Wes Smith. His gift for taking boring medical speak and converting it into a factual but easy-to-read narrative is truly exceptional.

The book was long a dream for me but it became a reality thanks to a chance conversation with dynamic literary agent Jan Miller of Dupree-Miller & Associates. Nena Madonia, a DMA literary agent, also was essential to this project. I am grateful also to Rodale Inc. and its team of editors including vice president Colin Dickerman, editorial assistant Gena Smith, senior project editor Nancy N. Bailey, and copy editor Patty Fernandez. We are grateful for their support, guidance, and hard work on this demanding project.

Finally, I would like to thank all of the employees at the Colorado Center for Reproductive Medicine, who made it possible for me to complete this book and who endeavor every day to make life better for our patients.

In serving our patients, physicians often spend far too many hours away from their families. This book demanded even more of my time, so I have dedicated it to my family, Cheri, Beau, and Michael. Without their love, support, and understanding, I could not have accomplished this task. Thanks.

INDEX

Underscored page references indicate sidebars and tables. **Boldface** references indicate illustrations.